TABLE OF CONTENTS

Introduction
- Benefits of Noom
- Promotes behavioral changes
- Foods to eat and avoid
- Noom Diet One-week sample menu
- Noom Diet Meal prep recipes for weight loss
- NOOM RECIPES FOR WEIGHT LOSS
- Slow Grilled Chinese Char Siu Chicken
- Vegan parmesan cheese (optional)
- Easy Creamy Cajun Shrimp Pasta
- Healthy Chicken Taco Soup
- Caribbean Steamed Fish
- Crispy Potato Tacos
- Baked Salmon Cake Balls With Rosemary Aioli
- Crispy Baked Falafel

Easy Vegetable Stirfry With Peanut Sauce
- Grilled Chicken and Vegetable Shish Kebabs
- Vegan Chorizo Tostadas
- Noom Easy Baked BBQ Seitan
- Noom Slow Cooker Jamaican Chicken Stew
- Noom Crockpot Beef Vegetable Soup
- Mexican Stuffed Peppers
- Honey Mustard Chicken with Brussel Sprouts

Mexican Salad with Chipotle Shrimp
One-Pot Chicken Soup with White Beans & Kale
Chicken and Zucchini Stir Fry
Noom Spicy Tuna Poke Bowls
Blackened Chicken Cobb Salad
. Chipotle Chicken Tostadas with Pineapple Salsa
Creamy Chipotle Sweet Potato Penne Pasta
Rosemary Citrus One Pan Baked Salmon
Arroz Con Pollo, Lightened Up
Instant Pot Beef and Barley Stew
Smashed Pea and Ricotta Pappardelle
White Bean and Tuna Salad with Basil Vinaigrette
Chicago-Style Chicken Dogs
Cheesy Tex-Mex Stuffed Chicken
. Red Curry Shrimp and Cilantro Rice
Noom Loaded Spaghetti
Bow Ties with Spring Vegetables
Pizza Party
Chicken with Cheesy Broccoli Soup
Zesty Tofu and Quinoa
Noom Pork with Roasted Vegetables
Seared Scallops with Lemon Juice and Sage
Shrimp and Broccoli Pasta Salad
Shaved Zucchini Salad
Jalapeño-Watermelon Salad
Spaghetti and Meatballs
Eggplant and Zucchini Lasagna

INTRODUCTION

Noom aims to help you lose weight like most commercial diet plans and programs — by creating a calorie deficit.

A calorie deficit occurs when you consistently consume fewer calories than you burn each day

Noom estimates your daily calorie needs based on your gender, age, height, weight, and your answers to a series of lifestyle questions.

Depending on your goal weight and timeframe, Noom uses an algorithm to estimate how many calories you need to eat each day. This is known as your calorie budget.

For safety reasons and to ensure adequate nutrition, the app does not allow a daily calorie budget below 1,200 calories for women or 1,400 calories for men

Noom encourages food logging and daily weigh-ins — two self-monitoring behaviors associated with weight loss and long-term weight loss maintenance

Can it help you lose weight?

Any reduced-calorie diet plan or program can help you lose weight if you follow it

Still, sticking with a diet is difficult for many people. Most diets fail because they're difficult to maintain

To date, no studies have compared the effectiveness of Noom with other weight loss diets, but researchers have analyzed data from Noom users.

In one study in nearly 36,000 Noom users, 78% experienced weight loss while they were using the app for an average of 9 months, with 23% experiencing more than a 10% loss, compared with their starting weight

The study also found that those who tracked their diet and weight more frequently were more successful in losing weight

BENEFITS OF NOOM

Noom's program emphasizes a long-term approach to weight loss. It may have several benefits over quick-fix methods.

Focuses on calorie and nutrient density

Noom emphasizes calorie density, a measure of how many calories a food or beverage provides relative to its weight or volume.

The program categorizes foods into a color system — green, yellow, and red — based on their calorie density and concentration of nutrients.

Foods with the lowest calorie density, highest concentration of nutrients, or both, are considered green. Foods with the highest calorie density, lowest concentration of nutrients, or both, are labeled red, while yellow foods fall in between.

Calorie-dense foods contain a large number of calories in a small amount of food, whereas items of low calorie density have fewer calories in a large amount of food

Generally, low-calorie-dense foods, such as fruits and vegetables, contain more water and fiber and are low in fat.

On the other hand, high-calorie-dense foods, such as fatty fish, meats, nut butters, sweets, and desserts, typically provide fat or added sugars but lack water and fiber.

Diets comprised mainly of low-calorie-dense foods and

beverages are associated with less hunger, weight loss, and risk of chronic conditions like heart disease than diets rich in high-calorie-dense foods

No food is off limits

Several popular diets can be restricting by limiting certain foods or entire food groups. This can promote disordered eating or obsessive behaviors surrounding healthy or "clean" eating

Noom takes the opposite approach, offering flexibility by allowing all foods to fit into your diet.

Because some high-calorie-dense foods like nuts contain important nutrients, and completely eliminating desserts and other treats is neither realistic nor worthwhile, Noom doesn't forbid these items but encourages less of them.

The program does this to help you stay within or near your daily calorie budget.

Noom's library of recipes also helps you determine which foods and recipes are appropriate for you based on any food allergies or intolerances you may have.

PROMOTES BEHAVIORAL CHANGES

Losing weight and leading a healthy lifestyle goes beyond what and how much you eat.

It's also about forming new healthy behaviors, reinforcing the healthy habits you already have, and breaking any unhealthy patterns that sabotage your goals

Without behavioral change, any weight lost with a reduced-calorie diet tends to be regained over time — often in excess of what was initially lost

In fact, in a review of 29 long-term weight loss studies, people gained back 33% of their initial weight loss at 1 year, on average, and 79% after 5 years

Recognizing that behavioral change is difficult, Noom uses a psychology-based curriculum that encourages self-efficacy — the belief in your ability to execute habits necessary to reach your goals

In this way, Noom may better equip you with the tools and education necessary for effective behavioral change that underlies successful long-term weight loss maintenance.

Indeed, one study found that 78% of nearly 36,000 Noom users sustained their weight loss over 9 months. It's unclear whether weight loss is sustained after this time

Cons and other factors to consider

While Noom is an excellent, comprehensive tool you can use to help you reach your health goals, there are a few things to keep in mind about the app.

Keep in mind that tracking your food and calorie intake, whether through Noom or another program, may promote disordered eating patterns. These may include food anxiety and excessive calorie restriction

However, if you're employed by a company that offers a workplace health and wellness program, speak with your company's human resources department. You might receive a financial incentive to participate in wellness programs like Noom.

However, you may prefer face-to-face rather than virtual coaching sessions. If this is the case, you might intentionally limit or avoid communication with Noom's health coaches and thus not experience the program's full weight loss benefits.

In fact, two studies in people with prediabetes showed that higher engagement with coaches and educational articles in the Noom app was significantly associated with weight loss

FOODS TO EAT AND AVOID

Noom categorizes food as green, yellow, or red based on its calorie and nutrient density.

The app recommends consuming a set percentage of foods from each color — 30% green, 45% yellow, and 25% red.

Green

Fruits: bananas, apples, strawberries, watermelon, blueberries

Vegetables: tomatoes, cucumbers, salad greens, carrots, onions, spinach

Starchy vegetables: parsnips, beets, sweet potatoes, squash

Diary: skim milk, non-fat yogurt, non-fat Greek yogurt, non-fat cheese sticks

Dairy alternatives: unsweetened almond, cashew, or soy milk

Whole grains: oatmeal, brown rice, whole-grain bread, whole-grain pita, whole-grain pasta, whole-grain tortilla, whole-grain cereals

Condiments: marinara, salsa, sauerkraut, ketchup, light mayo

Beverages: unsweetened tea and coffee

Yellow

Lean meats: grilled chicken, turkey, and lean cuts of beef, pork, and lamb

Seafood: tuna, salmon, tilapia, scallops

Dairy: low-fat milk, low-fat cheeses, low-fat cottage cheese, Greek yogurt

Legumes and seeds: lentils, pinto beans, chickpeas, peas, quinoa, black beans, soy beans

Grains and grain products: couscous, white rice, white bread, white pasta

Beverages: diet soda, beer

Red

Meats: ham, red meats, fried meats, bacon, sausage, hot dogs, hamburgers

Nuts and nut butters: peanut butter, almond butter, almonds, walnuts

Desserts and sweets: cake, chocolate, cookies, candy, pastries

Snack foods: french fries, potato chips, energy and snack bars

Condiments and toppings: butter, mayonnaise, ranch dressing

Beverages: wine, juices like orange juice

NOOM DIET ONE-WEEK SAMPLE MENU

This meal plan would not apply to everyone since calorie recommendations are individualized, but it provides a general overview of the foods included from the green, yellow, and red categories.

Monday

Breakfast: raspberry yogurt parfait

Lunch: vegetarian barley soup

Dinner: fennel, orange, and arugula salad

Snack: creamy cucumber and dill salad

Tuesday

Breakfast: banana-ginger smoothie

Lunch: roasted orange tilapia and asparagus

Dinner: mushroom and rice soup

Snack: deviled eggs

Wednesday

Breakfast: vegetable skillet frittata

Lunch: broccoli quinoa pilaf

Dinner: pork lettuce wraps

Snack: homemade yogurt pops

Thursday

Breakfast: egg sandwich

Lunch: chicken and avocado pita pockets

Dinner: pasta with shellfish and mushrooms

Snack: mixed nuts

Friday

Breakfast: spinach-tomato frittata

Lunch: salmon with tabbouleh salad

Dinner: grilled chicken with corn salsa

Snack: chocolate cake

Saturday

Breakfast: banana-apple and nut oatmeal

Lunch: turkey cheddar tacos

Dinner: green bean casserole

Snack: hummus and peppers

Sunday

Breakfast: scrambled egg wrap

Lunch: loaded spinach salad

Dinner: salmon patties with green beans

Snack: cream cheese fruit dip with apples

Healthy meal prep ideas for weight loss

Planning your meals ahead of time will help you:

Save time preparing food

Save money on restaurant meals / fast food

Stick to your calorie budget

Make healthier food choices

Enjoy your favorite foods in moderation

As such, meal prep is one of the key ingredients in any weight loss equation.

What is meal prep?

Meal prep is exactly what is sounds like! Planning and preparing meals ahead of time. Let's be real, even if you love cooking at home, time is typically the limiting factor. Not only can meal prep help save you time and money, it can also help ensure you have healthy choices that allow you to continue working towards those goals to lose weight!

Another benefit of meal prepping is the fact that it helps you develop awareness around the choices you are making. Spending time planning, shopping, and preparing meals is far more of a commitment than ordering from the cafeteria or going through the drive-thru. This commitment can ensure that your choices are both delicious and align with your health goals!

How do I budget calories for my meal plan?

Meal prep for weight loss

Although meal prep may look different depending on your goals, planning your calories for each meal is vital when using meal prep for weight loss. A simple way to plan your calorie needs per meal is to simply divide your daily calories by the number of meals you want to eat in a day!

Let's break down how to plan for a days worth of meals! Say your budget for the day is 1700 calories.

To get your calorie range for each meal, simply divide 1700 by the number of meals and snacks you want to eat in a day, let's say 3 meals and 2 snacks. This would break down to around 500 calories for breakfast, lunch, and dinner and 100 calories per snack.

Once you have a calorie range for each meal and snack, plan out meals that fall into these calorie ranges. Not sure how to determine calories in a meal? This is where the Noom app comes into play! Logging via the Noom app can be a great way to develop awareness around caloric density and to learn how many calories your planned meals have.

Once you have this information, you can easily find recipes to cook ahead of time for each day. Wanting to know how to use this information to meal prep for the entire week? We got you covered.

How should I store my prepared meals?

Weekly meal prep

After determining your calorie goal per meal, and finding recipes that you enjoy (don't worry, those are yet to come), make sure you are set up with enough microwave-safe containers that can easily store your food for the week! These containers not only help with portion control but also make it super easy to grab them and go.

When choosing recipes and food options for your meal prep, it is a good idea to consider your time frame and how you will store your food. The Food Safety and Inspection Service of the USDA recommends cooked meat should be consumed within

3-5 days of being prepared and be reheated to an internal temp of 165 degrees. On the flip side, salads and veggies that will be eaten cold should be kept at a temperature under 40 degrees. Don't have a fridge at work? It might be a good idea to invest in a cooler lunchbox to keep you healthy and enjoying those delicious meals you worked so hard preparing!

After getting your specific calories planned out and your containers ready to go, it's time to make a list and head to the grocery store! How do you know what goes on that list? By finding healthy and delicious recipes! We have compiled a list of some of our favorite meal prep recipes for weight loss, below!

NOOM DIET MEAL PREP RECIPES FOR WEIGHT LOSS

Breakfast

Overnight oats: A simple and easy prep for delicious oats that are flavorful and give you a boost of energy to start your day!

Egg Cups: A staple meal prep breakfast, egg cups let you pick your favorite ingredients and create a high protein morning meal.

Bacon egg and Kale breakfast salad: Salad for breakfast? You bet! This salad gives you a perfect balance of green, yellow, and red and helps you start your day on the right foot!

Salads your meal prep style?

Snacks

Coconut energy balls: A lower sugar alternative to protein bars, these energy balls give you a serving of protein and fat to help keep you energized!

Hard-boiled egg + fruit: Boil eggs ahead of time for a quick and protein packed snack! What's the trick to easily peeling your hard-boiled eggs? Start with a pot of boiling water and drop your eggs straight from the fridge! Boil for about 10 minutes and place right into an ice bath. Trust us, the shell practically falls off!

Hummus + veggies: A match made in heaven, hummus makes the perfect pair to any of your favorite in-season veggies!

Lunch

Chicken, rice and broccoli bowl: Less adventurous when it comes to your meal prep? This chicken and rice bowl is simple and delicious.

Diggin' the chicken? Want more delicious chicken meal prep recipes? Check them out here!

Grilled romaine with cherry tomato salad: This grilled salad screams summer! It would also go great paired with your favorite protein!

Slow cooker vegetable and lentil soup: Set it and forget it, the more your style when it comes to cooking? Give this slow cooker veggies soup a peak!

Crucial tip: Keep prepared meals exciting

When it comes to healthy meal prep ideas it is important to remember the balance between enjoying your food and working towards your health goals! Let's be real, food is delicious! It is something to be enjoyed. Finding ways to make food taste good and also let you work towards your weight loss goals vital to successful long term meal prep!

How do you do this? By trying new recipes and finding what you enjoy! We always like trying at least one new recipe a week to mix things up, keep it fresh, and find our favorites! You will be amazed at the benefit meal prep provides to your daily food choices and your journey to lose weight!

How can I save money with meal prep?

Loving these recipes and our strategies to meal prep? Us too! Worried about breaking the bank? Don't be! Although grocery shopping can be more challenging when on a strict budget, quality meal prep doesn't have to be expensive! In fact, preparing your meals for the week can often be more affordable than daily meals out.

NOOM RECIPES FOR WEIGHT LOSS

Slow Cooker Seafood Ramen

Ingredients:

64 oz broth (seafood, vegetable, or chicken

4–6 oz ramen

1 lb seafood

2 green onions, sliced

2 tbsp low-sodium soy sauce

2 tbsp rice vinegar

2 garlic cloves, minced

1/4 cup kale, chopped

1/2 lb tomatoes, sliced

1/4 tsp sesame oil

1 tsp salt

1/4 tsp pepper

1/8 tsp red pepper flakes

Directions:

Add all ingredients except the seafood, kale and ramen to the slow cooker. Stir to mix well.

Cook on high for 2-3 hours, or low for 4-6 hours.

Add seafood, kale & ramen and cook for an additional 15-30 minutes.

Per Serving: 250 calories, 2.7 g fat (0.3 g sat), 29.5 g protein, 27 g carb, 2588.3 mg sodium, 3.9 g sugars, 1.7 g fiber

Turkey Carrot Mushroom Dumplings

Ingredients:

3/4 c. carrots finely julienned

1 lb ground turkey

1/2 c. mushrooms finely chopped

2 tsp soy sauce

1 tsp rice wine

1 tsp sesame oil

1/2 tsp onion powder

1/8 tsp salt

2 tsp cornstarch

30 dumpling wrappers

Directions:

Put carrots in a microwavable bowl and cover with water. Cook until tender, about 3 minutes depending on how finely shredded the carrots are. Drain and let cool.

In a large bowl, mix together cooked carrots, turkey, mushrooms, soy sauce, rice wine, sesame oil, onion powder, salt and cornstarch. Stir together until well combined.

Spoon a well rounded teaspoon of filling onto a dumpling wrapper. Seal filling with wrapper. Wrap remaining dumplings.

Bring water to boil in the bottom of the steamer pot. Place dumplings in a parchment paper lined steamer. Steam 15 minutes until cooked through.

Per serving: 48 calories, 1 g fat (0 g sat), 3 g protein, 4 g carb, 87 mg sodium

SLOW GRILLED CHINESE CHAR SIU CHICKEN

Ingredients:

1/4 c. organic brown sugar

1/4 c. raw honey

1/4 c. organic ketchup

1/4 c. gluten-free soy sauce

3 Tbsp beet powder

2 Tbsp rice vinegar

1 Tbsp gluten-free hoisin sauce

1/2 tsp Chinese five-spice powder

Sea salt and freshly ground black pepper to taste

2 1/2 lbs boneless skinless chicken thighs

Cooking oil spray

Directions:

In a large bowl, mix together brown sugar, honey, ketchup, soy sauce, beet powder, vinegar, hoisin sauce, five-spice powder, salt and pepper.

Add chicken and toss well, coating all the pieces well; cover and refrigerate for two days to marinate.

Heat grill; spray cooking oil on grates; grill chicken until cooked through, about 10 minutes per side.

Per serving: 328 calories, 8 g fat (2 g sat), 38 g protein, 25 g carb, 845 mg sodium, 24 g sugars, 1 g fiber

Creamy Kabocha Squash and Roasted Red Pepper Pasta

Ingredients:

1/2 c. raw cashews

1 small kabocha squash

1 head of garlic

1/3 cauliflower, cut into large florets

1/2 medium onion (roughly chopped)

1 stalk celery, roughly chopped

1 medium carrot, roughly chopped

1/4 c. roasted red peppers, drained

2 Tbsp nutritional yeast

Optional: A pinch red pepper flakes

2 to 3 c. vegetable broth (or as needed)

Salt and black pepper, to taste

1/2 to 3/4 c. fresh basil (unpacked), sliced

2 lb gluten-free spaghetti noodles (or pasta of your choice)

Serve with:

VEGAN PARMESAN CHEESE (OPTIONAL)

Fresh basil, sliced

Black pepper

Directions:

Soak the cashews in water overnight. If you do not have time to, you can also bring a small pot of water to a boil, remove it from heat and add in the cashews. Allow them to soak until you blend the sauce together (which will be about 1 hour).

Preheat the oven to 400°F and position the rack to the middle of the oven. Line a baking sheet with parchment paper or a silicone mat. Wash and dry the kabocha squash, place it (whole) on the baking sheet and into the oven for 18-20 minutes. Remove the pan from the oven and cool until the squash is easy to handle. If the stem of it is protruding, use a knife to carefully remove it. Slice the squash in half vertically, then scoop out the seeds and fiber using a spoon. Slice the squash into 1-inch wedges, trying to keep the slices uniform for even cooking. Place 6 or 7 the slices of the cooked squash (roughly 1 1/2 cups) onto your lined baking sheet. The remaining kabocha squash can be cooked on an additional baking sheet with the same baking time and directions below. It can be stored in the fridge in an airtight container for up to a week.

Using your hands, remove loose skin from the outside of the

head of garlic. With a sharp knife, cut 1/4"-inch off the top of the garlic, or enough to expose the tops of the cloves. Place the garlic head (cut side down) onto the baking sheet along with the cauliflower florets, onions, celery, and carrots. Sprinkle with salt and pepper and place back into the oven for 40 minutes, flipping/mixing halfway through.

10 minutes before the vegetables are done, prepare the pasta.

Once you have removed the baking sheet from the oven, allow the veggies to cool until easily handled and then use a knife to carefully remove the skin from the kabocha and add it into a high speed blender. You can discard this or snack on it as you continue cooking. Using you hands, squeeze the soften garlic cloves out of the head and into the blender, along with the soaked cashews (drained), the remaining vegetables on the baking sheet, the roasted red peppers, nutritional yeast, red pepper flakes, 2 cups of vegetable broth plus salt and pepper as desired. Blend until smooth, adding as much of the additional 1 cup of vegetable broth as needed to thin out the sauce. Adjust seasonings to taste and then add in the sliced basil. Pulse the basil in until well combined (do not blend it as it will turn the sauce a weird color).

Drain the pasta, add it back into the pot and pour over the sauce. Mix until well combined.

Serve with a sprinkle of fresh parmesan, basil and black pepper. Enjoy!

Per serving: 501 calories, 5.9 g fat (0 g sat), 17.8 g protein, 93.4 g carb, 56.3 mg sodium, 5.8 g sugars

Loaded Cauliflower

Ingredients:

1.25 lb cauliflower head, cut into florets

6 green onion, chopped into the green and white parts

2 tbsp butter

3 garlic cloves, minced

2 oz cream cheese

1/2 tsp sea salt

1/4 tsp black pepper

1.5 tsp ranch seasoning Mix, optional

3/4 c. organic heavy whipping cream

2 c. cheddar cheese, grated

4 slices sugar-free bacon, crumbled

Olive oil for roasting the cauliflower

Dollops of sour cream, optional

Directions:

Preheat the oven to 425 degrees.

Toss the cauliflower with ~2 Tbsp of olive oil then add it to a baking sheet. Roast the cauliflower on a baking sheet for 25 minutes. The cauliflower will get tender and some parts will brown up.

While the cauliflower is roasting, make the cheese sauce: Add butter, the white parts of the green onions, and the garlic cloves to a skillet on medium heat. Sauté until the onions are translucent (~3 minutes).

Add heavy cream, cream cheese, salt, ranch seasoning (if you're using it), and pepper to the skillet with the onions, garlic and butter. Turn the heat to medium low and continue to cook until the cream cheese is melted. Stir in 1.5 cups of the cheddar cheese to finish the cheese sauce.

Mix the cheese sauce and the roasted cauliflower, then add it to a baking dish. Top it with the remaining cheddar cheese and roast for an additional 20 minutes, or until the cauliflower is tender.

Top the baked cauliflower, with some dollops of sour cream, the green parts of the green onions, and the crumbled bacon.

Per serving: 315 calories, 28 g fat (17 g sat), 11 g protein, 5 g carb, 587 mg sodium, 2 g sugars, 1 g fiber

EASY CREAMY CAJUN SHRIMP PASTA

Ingredients:

8 oz linguine pasta

2 tsp olive oil Divided into 1 teaspoon servings.

1 lb raw shrimp, deveined and shells removed.

1 Tbsp cajun seasoning divided into 1/2 Tbsp servings. You can also use creole seasoning.

4 oz andouille sausage Sliced into 1 inch pieces. You can use more if you like.

1/2 c. chopped red peppers

1/2 c. chopped green peppers

1/2 c. chopped yellow or white onions

1 c. fire roasted diced tomatoes Drained from a can.

1 Tbsp butter

1/2 c. heavy whipping cream

1/2 c. unsweetened almond milk

4 oz cream cheese Cut into chunks.

1/2 c. shredded Parmesan Reggiano Cheese

Directions

Cook the pasta as per package instructions.

Place the shrimp in a bowl along with 1/2 Tbsp of cajun or creole seasoning. Mix to ensure the shrimp is fully coated.

Heat a skillet or pan on medium high heat. I use a cast iron skillet. Add 1 teaspoon of olive oil to the pan.

When hot, add the shrimp to the pan. Cook for 2-3 minutes on each side until it turns bright pink. Remove the shrimp and set aside.

Add an additional teaspoon of olive oil to the pan along with the chopped sausage, onions, green peppers, and red peppers.

Saute for 3-4 minutes until the vegetables are soft and the onions are translucent and fragrant. Remove the vegetables from the pan and set aside.

Reduce the heat on the pan to medium. Add the butter to the pan and allow it to melt.

Add in the heavy cream, almond milk, cream cheese, the remaining 1/2 tablespoon of cajun or creole seasoning, and parmesan reggiano cheese.

Continue to stir the sauce until all of the cheese has fully melted. The cream cheese may take some time to melt. Add in the fire roasted tomatoes and stir. Allow the mixture to cook for 2 minutes.

Add the shrimp, sausage, vegetables, and pasta to the pan and stir. Allow the pasta to cook for 4-5 minutes until combined. Serve.

Per serving: 384 calories, 28 g fat, 7 g protein, 22 g carb

HEALTHY CHICKEN TACO SOUP

Ingredients:

½ Tbsp avocado or coconut oil

1 small yellow onion, diced

1 small red bell pepper, diced

1 small green bell pepper, diced

5 cloves garlic, minced

1 lb boneless, skinless chicken breast

1 1/2 tsp salt (plus more to taste)

1 tsp dried oregano

1 tsp chipotle powder

1 tsp paprika

2 tsp cumin

¼ tsp black pepper

1 – 15 oz can fire roasted diced tomatoes

2 – 4.5 oz cans green chilies

¼ c. fresh lime juice

32 oz chicken broth

Cilantro, for serving

Diced red onion, for serving

Lime wedges, for serving

Directions:

Heat a large pot over medium-high heat. Once hot, add in the avocado or coconut oil. Next, add the peppers, onion, and garlic to the pot. Saute for 3-4 minutes until the onions start to become translucent.

Add the chicken breast, canned tomatoes, canned green chilies, spices, lime juice, and chicken broth to the pot. Stir until well combined. Bring the soup to a rolling boil and then reduce the heat to a simmer. Allow the soup to simmer for 30 minutes or until the chicken is tender and easy to shred.

Transfer the chicken breast from the soup to a small bowl. Use two forks to shred the meat. Add the chicken back to the soup and stir until well combined. Serve the soup with fresh cilantro, diced red onion, and fresh lime wedges. Enjoy!

Per serving: 258 calories, 6.1 g fat (1 g sat), 30 g protein, 22.7 g carb, 1960.9 mg sodium, 10.1 g sugars, 5.1 g fiber

Quick and Easy Mongolian Beef

Ingredients:

1 lb flank steak thinly sliced against the grain

2 Tbsp cornstarch

2-4 Tbsp canola oil

1 yellow onion sliced

2 green onions chopped, green and white parts separated

4 garlic cloves chopped

1-inch ginger chopped

¼ c. low sodium soy sauce

¼ c. water

1 Tbsp hoisin sauce

3 Tbsp brown sugar

Salt to taste

Directions:

Cover the flank steak with cornstarch, making sure each piece is covered. Set aside.

Heat the canola oil in a large skillet over medium-high heat. Once the oil is hot, add the flank steak to the frying pan in a single layer, making sure that the pieces are not touching. Cook for 1-2 minutes per side until each side is browned. Cook in batches until all the flank steak is cooked. Set aside.

Add sliced yellow onion, whites of green onions, garlic, and ginger to the skillet and stir fry for about 3 minutes, until the onions are slightly softened but still have a little crunch. Add soy sauce, water, hoisin sauce, and brown sugar and stir. Add steak back to the pan along with the green parts of the onions. Remove from heat and serve.

Per serving: 303 calories, 13 g fat (3 g sat), 26 g protein, 20 g carb, 670 mg sodium, 11 g sugars, 1 g fiber

CARIBBEAN STEAMED FISH

Ingredients:

2 lbs fish (porgy or snapper), cleaned and scaled

Juice of 1 lime

½ tsp black pepper

1 tsp salt

3 cloves garlic – 2 sliced and 1 crushed

About 15 sprigs thyme

½ Tbsp butter

½ Tbsp oil

2 carrots, thinly sliced

1 red pepper, thinly sliced

1 green pepper, thinly sliced

1 onion, thinly sliced

12 okra, ends cut off

1 hot pepper (scotch bonnet, habanero or wiri wiri), seeds removed

1 ½ cup water

Directions:

Season the fish with lime juice, crushed garlic, black pepper, salt and half of the thyme and set aside.

In a large, wide heavy bottom pot over medium heat, add oil and butter. When butter has melted, sauté carrots, red and green pepper, and onion until it has softened, about 5 minutes.

Add garlic slices and pepper and cook for just a minute or two. Add water and bring to a boil. Add fish to the pot. Spoon some of the vegetables on top of the fish. Add okra and the rest of the thyme.

Cover the pot and lower the heat to simmer then cook for 15 minutes until the fish is done. Remove from heat and serve.

Per serving: 378 calories, 7.4 g fat (1.2 g sat), 60.5 g protein, 13.1 g carb, 794 mg sodium, 5.5 g sugars, 3.3 g fiber

Corn Chowder Con Chile Poblano

Ingredients:

2 Tbsp vegetable oil

1 poblano pepper without seeds and thinly sliced

1 medium onion sliced

2 cloves of garlic roughly chopped

5 corn husks

4 medium potatoes cubed

1 tsp of salt

To serve:

Corn kernels

Pumpkin seeds

Cilantro microgreens or chopped cilantro

Olive oil

Freshly ground pepper

Directions:

In a large pot add the oil and the sliced poblano chile. Leave it there until it begins to soften. Add the onion and garlic. Leave for five more minutes or until you see that the onion is translucent.

Add the corn kernels, potatoes, salt and cover with water, add the salt and cover. Leave for 10-15 minutes or until the vegetables are cooked.

With a ladle, add about one-third of the vegetables and liquid into the container of a blender. Blend until fully liquefied and well integrated. Return to the pot with the rest of the vegetables. If you need more liquid, add a little more water. Check for seasoning and adjust if necessary.

Serve with a drizzle of olive oil, pumpkin seeds, corn kernels, sprouts or chopped cilantro. Finish with sea salt and pepper.

Per serving: 135 calories, 4 g fat (3 g sat), 4 g protein, 20 g carb, 403 mg sodium, 1 g sugars, 4 g fiber

CRISPY POTATO TACOS

Ingredients:

12 corn tortillas

1 c. mashed potatoes

4 Tbsp of vegetable oil or avocado oil

4 long wooden skewers

To serve:

Thinly sliced romaine lettuce or green cabbage

Radishes thinly sliced

Cilantro

Guacamole

Salsa verde

Directions:

Heat tortillas on a skillet for 10-15 seconds to make them pliable.

Put a spoonful of mashed potatoes in the center of each tortilla and spread it along the tortilla. Roll the tortilla and put it on a long skewer. Repeat until you put three or four tacos on the skewer.

Repeat with all the tortillas.

In a frying pan over high heat put a tablespoon of oil and put three or four tacos, leave until golden brown, three to five minutes, turn and brown on the other side.

Take out the tacos and put in a dish with a paper towel to absorb the excess oil.

Repeat until all the tacos are done.

To serve, put the crispy potato tacos on a plate and finish with the toppings. Enjoy immediately.

Per serving: 347 calories, 16 g fat (2 g sat), 6 g protein, 47 g carb, 51 mg sodium, 1 g sugars, 6 g fiber

Black Garlic, Sesame and Shitake Cod

Ingredients:

2 Alaskan Cod filets, frozen

1 clove black garlic

2 Tbsp olive oil

1 tsp sesame seeds

1/2 c. dried shiitake, rehydrated

Directions:

Preheat your oven to 450F.

Rinse frozen fish, pat dry with a paper towel, and place on a nonstick pan.

In a small bowl, place black garlic and warm in the microwave for 10 seconds.

Mash the garlic clove and add olive oil and sesame seeds.

Brush this mixture on frozen filets and sprinkle the mushrooms around the fish.

Place in the oven for 12-15 minutes, depending on the thickness of the fish. If your filets are on the thick side, flip halfway through cooking.

Serve alongside rice, your favorite salad, or whole grain.

Per serving: 241 calories, 15.8 g fat (2.1 g sat), 20.9 g protein, 6.1 g carb, 72 mg sodium, 1.3 g sugars, 1 g fiber

Shrimp Lettuce Wraps

Ingredients:

1 head butter lettuce or romaine lettuce hearts

¼ c. low-sodium chicken broth

1 Tbsp hoisin sauce

½ Tbsp low-sodium soy sauce

1 tsp rice vinegar

¼ tsp Asian sesame oil

1 1/2 tsp chili garlic sauce

½ tsp cornstarch

1 Tbsp canola or avocado oil divided

30 grams cashews little less than ¼ cup, coarsely chopped

6 oz shrimp deveined & cut into small cubes

1 large garlic clove minced

1/2 large red bell pepper seeded and diced

3 green onions the white and green parts, sliced

? c. chopped cilantro

1 carrot shredded or cut into thin strips

Directions:

Divide the lettuce into leaves and set aside.

In a small bowl, whisk together the chicken broth, hoisin sauce, soy sauce, rice vinegar, sesame oil, chili garlic sauce, and cornstarch. Set aside.

In a medium skillet, heat ½ Tbsp canola or avocado oil over medium-high heat until almost smoking.

Add the shrimp and stir-fry until browned. About 2 minutes. Transfer the shrimp to a plate and discard any juices from the pan.

In the same skillet, heat the other ½ tablespoon of oil over medium-high heat.

Add the garlic, bell pepper, green onions, and carrots.

Stir fry until tender-crisp, about 2 minutes.

Return the shrimp to the pan and add the cashews and cilantro. Add the soy-sauce mixture and stir-fry until the shrimp is thoroughly cooked. About 3 minutes.

Spoon the shrimp mixture evenly onto lettuce leaves.

Per serving: 269 calories, 14 g fat (2 g sat), 26 g protein, 17 g carb, 753 mg sodium, 7 g sugars, 3 g fiber

BAKED SALMON CAKE BALLS WITH ROSEMARY AIOLI

Ingredients:

2 lbs wild salmon fillets

1 tsp sea salt

1 tsp black pepper

1/2 medium purple onion, chopped

1/2 c. organic spinach, chopped

1/2 red bell pepper, diced

1/2 yellow red pepper, diced

1 small jalapeño, diced

2/3 c. breadcrumbs

1-2 Tbsps Old Bay seasoning

1/2 c. fresh parsley, chopped

1/3 c. vegan Mayo

1/2 c. dijon mustard

1 large organic egg, room temp.

4 Tbsps lemon juice

1-2 Tbsps sriracha sauce

1/2 c. vegan mayo

4 tsp lemon juice

2 garlic cloves, crushed + minced

1/4 tsp sea salt

2 sprigs fresh rosemary, chopped

Directions:

First, preheat the oven to 400 degrees Fahrenheit.

Season salmon with sea salt + black pepper and roast on a baking sheet (lined with parchment paper) for about 20 minutes, or until cooked through.

Once cooked, remove from the oven and set aside while it cools for 5 minutes before shredding or flaking into medium chunks.

Meanwhile, add onions, bell peppers, jalapeños, spinach, old bay seasoning, breadcrumbs, parsley, mayo, dijon mustard, egg, sriracha and lemon juice to a large bowl. Then add shredded salmon and mix all ingredients together, using your hands.

Scoop about 2 Tbsps of batter and form into a ball with your hands and line on a baking sheet (lined with parchment paper). Repeat until all batter is used.

Bake salmon balls for 15-20 minutes, or until slightly crisp and golden brown.

Combine vegan mayo, lemon juice, garlic cloves, sea salt, and rosemary in a medium bowl and whisk together thoroughly. Refrigerate for aioli until ready to use.

Per serving: 173 calories, 6.7 g fat (1.6 g sat), 20.5 g protein, 8.6 g carb, 6011 mg sodium, 3.3 g sugars, 1.2 g fiber

CRISPY BAKED FALAFEL

Ingredients:

1 c. dried chickpeas, soaked in water overnight

1/2 c. fresh parsley

1/2 medium onion chopped

3 garlic cloves chopped

1 tsp cumin

1 tsp coriander

1/4 tsp black pepper

1 tsp salt

1/4 c. vegetable oil

Directions:

Preheat the oven to 400F.

Once the chickpeas are done soaking, drain them and rinse with fresh water.

Add the soaked chickpeas, parsley, onion, garlic, spices, pepper and salt to a food processor. Pulse a few times, until you have a consistent, coarse texture.

Create 10-12 small falafel balls with your hands.

In a medium pan, heat the vegetable oil on the stovetop, and add the falafel balls. I recommend you do this in 2 batches.

Cook the falafel balls in the oil for 2 minutes on each side, using a spatula to carefully flip over. Once done, add them to a parchment paper-lined baking dish.

Once all the falafels are cooked on the pan and added to the baking dish, drizzle the remaining oil from the pan onto the falafels, and bake for 20 minutes or until browned and crisp. Flip halfway with a spatula.

Enjoy with pita, greens, rice, or your favorite pairings.

Per serving: 128 calories, 6.7 g fat (1.2 g sat), 4.1 g protein, 13 g carb, 261 mg sodium, 2.4 g sugars, 3.7 g fiber

EASY VEGETABLE STIRFRY WITH PEANUT SAUCE

Ingredients:

Peanut Sauce:

1 Tbsp sesame oil

1/2 tsp ground ginger (1 tbsp fresh)

1/4 tsp garlic powder (2 cloves)

1/2 c. smooth unsweetened peanut butter

3 Tbsp low sodium soy sauce

2 Tbsp freshly squeezed lime juice

2 Tbsp maple syrup

2 Tbsp fresh lime juice

1 Tbsp rice vinegar

1/4 cc-1/3 cc water as needed

Optional: Sriracha, to taste

Stirfy:

6 oz dried noodles of choice (see notes)

1 Tbsp cooking oil of choice

3 cloves garlic, finely minced

2 Tbsp green onions sliced

1 Tbsp freshly grated ginger

1/3 c. shredded red cabbage

4 oz crimini mushrooms, sliced

1 medium carrot, thinly sliced

1 medium red bell pepper, thinly sliced

1 c. broccoli

2 large handfuls fresh baby spinach

Garnish:

Cilantro, finely chopped

Green onions, sliced

Toasted sesame seeds or crushed peanuts

1 large lime, sliced

Directions:

Prepare the peanut sauce: In a small pot over medium-low, add in the sesame oil, garlic and ginger. Cook until fragrant, about 2 minutes. Add in the remaining ingredients for the peanut sauce and whisk together until uniform. Allow the mixture to come to a low simmer and then remove from heat and set aside.

Prepare the noodles according to the package directions. Once the noodles are cooked, drain them, rinse under cold water, add them back into the cooking pot and toss them with about 1 teaspoon of sesame oil to prevent sticking.

In the meantime, set a large wok over medium heat. Add in the cooking oil along with the garlic, green onions and ginger. Sauté, stirring often, for 3 minutes or until fragrant.

Next add in the cabbage, mushrooms, carrots, bell pepper and broccoli. Cook for an additional 4 minutes.

Once the vegetables have cooked, add in the spinach, peanut sauce and cooked noodles. Mix until everything is well combined and cook for 1-2 minutes more, or until everything is warmed through.

Serve with a garnish of cilantro, green and toasted sesame seeds, plus an extra wedge of lime on the side. Enjoy!

Per serving: 388 calories, 19.7 g fat, 8.7 g protein, 47 g carb, 294.5 mg sodium, 11.6 g sugars

GRILLED CHICKEN AND VEGETABLE SHISH KEBABS

Ingredients:

2 Tbsp Better Than Bouillon roasted chicken base

2 lb boneless chicken breasts

8 oz cubed pineapples

1 red bell pepper

1 green bell pepper

1 orange bell pepper

1 whole zucchini

2 tsp oregano

2 tsp black pepper

2 tsp paprika

For the teriyaki pineapple sauce:

1/2 c. low-sodium soy sauce

2 tsp minced garlic

2 tsp Sesame Oil

2 Tbsp fresh pineapple juice

2 tsp cornstarch

1 tsp black pepper

1/4 tsp Himalayan salt

1/4 tsp garlic powder

2 Tbsp brown sugar

Directions:

Begin by starting your fire on the grill and allow the temperature to reach 350 degrees.

Cut your chicken breast into cubes and place into a large bowl. Season chicken with oregano, black pepper and paprika then rub ingredients into the chicken.

Add Better Than Bouillon roasted chicken base to the chicken. Mix together well then set to the side.

Remove the stem and seeds from each of the bell peppers and cut into large pieces. Chop the zucchini into slices.

Place each ingredient individually onto the skewers in desired order.

Place each chicken and veggie skewer onto the grill. Grill for 4 minutes each side. Remove from heat.

For the sauce, add all ingredients into a small cooking pan on medium/high heat until it begins to bubble then lower heat to simmer and cook for 8 minutes and remove from heat and allow to cool.

Serve immediately.

Per serving: 408 calories, 6 g fat (0.4 g sat), 56.7 g protein, 34 g carb, 1278 mg sodium, 24.2 g sugars, 3.9 g fiber

VEGAN CHORIZO TOSTADAS

Ingredients:

4 c. of shaved Brussels sprouts

2 Tbsp of vegetable oil

2 Tbsp of chili powder ground dried chili powder

1 tsp of garlic powder

1/2 tsp of ground cumin

1/4 tsp freshly pepper

1/8 tsp ground cinnamon

Pinch of ground cloves

1/2 tsp apple cider vinegar

1/2 tsp salt

12 corn tostada shells

1 c. refried beans

1 avocado sliced

Mexican crema (I use cashew cream)

Directions:

In a skillet over medium heat add the oil and the shaved Brussels sprouts.

Leave them until they are soft, like 3 minutes. Add all the species and mix well. Leave everything for 5 more minutes or until the Brussel sprouts begin to brown on the edges.

Be careful not to burn them. When ready, remove from heat and add the vinegar. Mix and set aside.

For putting together the tostadas add 2 tablespoons of refried black beans and spread them well throughout the tostada.

Then add three or four tablespoons of the powerful vegan chorizo, aka, the Brussel sprouts with Mexican spices.

Finish each tostada with slices of avocado and drizzle with cashew or tofu crema.

Per serving: 268 calories, 11 g fat (4 g sat), 7 g protein, 37 g carb, 314 mg sodium, 3 g sugars, 10 g fiber

NOOM EASY BAKED BBQ SEITAN

Ingredients:

1 c. vital wheat gluten

2 Tbsp nutritional yeast

1 tsp garlic powder

2 tsp smoked paprika

2 tsp onion powder

1 Tbsp soy sauce

2 Tbsp tahini

1 c. veggie broth

1/3 c. BBQ sauce of choice

Directions:

Preheat the oven to 350F.

In a mixing bowl, add in vital wheat gluten, nutritional yeast, garlic powder, smoked paprika, and onion powder then with a fork mix well to combine.

Add in soy sauce, tahini and vegetable broth, then with your fork, whisk to combine liquid into the flour until a dough like ball forms.

With your hands, gently knead the gluten ball a few times making sure not to over do it. Should take no more than a minute.

Transfer dough to a lined baking sheet. Flatten and spread dough out until it is half an inch thick.

Place the baking sheet in the oven for 20-25 minutes.

Remove seitan from the oven and brush both sides with your favorite BBQ sauce. At this stage you can either grill or rebake your seitan.

Place seitan back in the oven for another 10 minutes. You may also opt to broil on high for about 2-3 minutes to help give a little char to the ends of your seitan.

Place seitan on a preheated electric grill and allow to cook and sear for about 4-5 minutes on each side or until grill marks appear on the surface of the seitan.

Once seitan is cooked, place on a clean surface or plate to rest for 3-5 minutes, then cut and serve as desired.

Per serving: 138 calories, 4.6 g fat (0.6 g sat), 10 g protein, 15.6 g carb, 564 mg sodium, 4.8 g sugars, 2.5 g fiber

Aloo Gobi (Spiced Potato and Cauliflower)

Ingredients:

¼ c. grapeseed avocado, or other neutral oil

1 tsp cumin seeds

½ tsp nigella seeds – (kalonji) optional

1 medium onion finely chopped

5 garlic cloves crushed

3/4 inch piece ginger crushed

3 small to medium tomatoes finely chopped

2 tsp coriander powder

1 tsp cumin powder

1/2 tsp turmeric

¼ tsp red chili powder or more to taste

1 tsp salt or more to taste

1 small head cauliflower cut into small florets (about 1 lb or 500 grams chopped)

2 medium potatoes peeled and cut into 1/2-inch cubes (around 350 grams), and placed in a bowl of water to prevent browning

1 green chili pepper sliced or chopped

1/2 tsp soy sauce or tamari

1/4 tsp lemon or lime juice or to taste

2 Tbsp chopped cilantro leaves to garnish

Directions:

Heat oil in a non-stick pan over medium-high heat. Add the cumin and nigella seeds and let them sizzle for a few seconds. Add the chopped onions and sauté, stirring frequently, until they turn lightly golden, about 5-6 minutes.

Add the garlic and ginger and sauté until the raw smell disappears, about 30 seconds. Add the tomatoes, spice powders (coriander, cumin, turmeric, red chili) and salt. Cook until the tomatoes are soft and the oil begins to separate from them, about 4-5 minutes.

Add the potatoes, cauliflower, and green chili pepper. Stir-fry for about 4-5 minutes.

Turn the heat down to low-medium, cover, and let cook for about 20 minutes, stirring once or twice in between.

When the vegetables are cooked and all the moisture is gone, turn off the heat and add the soy sauce and lemon juice. Mix well and garnish with chopped cilantro. Serve with roti, naan, or rice.

Per serving: 164 calories, 2.5 g fat (0.5 g sat), 5.3 g protein, 29.8 g carb, 755 mg sodium, 7.1 g sugars, 7.4 g fiber

NOOM SLOW COOKER JAMAICAN CHICKEN STEW

Ingredients:

3 lb chicken parts

2 tsp curry powder

1 ½ tsp dried thyme

¾ tsp ground allspice

½ tsp red pepper flakes

½ tsp black pepper

½ tsp salt

2 tsp olive oil

1 medium onion chopped

3 cloves garlic minced

½ c. red wine

1 ½ c. 15 ounces black beans, rinsed and drained

1 ½ c. 15 ounces diced tomatoes, undrained

Directions:

Toss chicken with curry powder, thyme, allspice, red pepper flakes, black pepper and salt.

Heat oil in a large skillet. Add onions and garlic and sauté until onions are softened, about 3 minutes. Add chicken mixture to skillet and brown on both sides. Add wine and let cook for a few minutes. Add tomatoes and black beans and mix well. Transfer to crock pot and cook in high for 4-5 hours until tender and meat is falling off the bone. Alternatively, you can continue to cook the chicken on the stove top for about 25-30 minutes until chicken is done.

Per serving: 423 calories, 24 g fat (6 g sat), 32 g protein, 13 g carb, 557 mg sodium, 2 g sugars, 4 g fiber

Slow Roasted Salmon Citrus Salad

Ingredients:

½ red onion

2 Tbsp red wine vinegar

Boston lettuce leaves

1 avocado

Aleppo pepper flakes

3 roasted beets quartered

2 orange peeled, cut into segments

1 grapefruit peeled, cut into segments

1 large tomato halved, cut into ¼" thick slices

½ English cucumber sliced

1 lb Slow Roasted Citrus Salmon

Flakey salt such as fleur de sel or Maldon salt

Ingredients for the citrus shallot vinaigrette:

1 Tbsp shallot minced

2 Tbsp fresh lemon juice or orange juice

1 ½ tsp rice wine vinegar

1 garlic clove smashed

5 Tbsp extra virgin olive oil

Salt and pepper to taste

Directions:

Pickle onions by placing onion and vinegar in small bowl, and letting them sit for 15 minutes.

Meanwhile, line serving plate with lettuce leaves.

Cut avocado in half and remove pit. Scoop spoonfuls of avocado onto plate; season with flakey salt and aleppo pepper.

Arrange quartered beets on plate. Arrange orange and grapefruit segments on plate.

Lightly salt tomato slices. Place on plate.

Lightly salt cucumbers and place on plate.

Scatter pickled onions on plate.

Break salmon into pieces and arrange on plate.

Drizzle Citrus Shallot Vinaigrette on top and sprinkle with a little flakey salt to finish.

Per serving: 336 calories, 21 g fat (3 g sat), 17 g protein, 20 g carb, 70 mg sodium, 11 g sugars, 5 g fiber

Spicy Korean Beef Noodle Soup

Ingredients:

1.7 oz mung bean noodles (sometimes called cellophane or glass noodles)

1 c. cooked short rib meat shredded (from rich beef broth recipe)

2 Tbsp toasted sesame oil

1 ½ - 2 Tbsp Korean red pepper flakes

1 Tbsp garlic chopped

4 c. Rich Beef Broth

1 c. water

2 c. bok choy chopped

4 fresh shitake mushrooms sliced

2 scallions cut into 2" lengths

Extra Korean red pepper flakes for serving

Fish sauce or soy sauce for serving

Directions:

Soak mung bean noodles in hot water for 20-30 minutes; drain.

Heat sesame oil, red pepper flakes and garlic in a small pan until fragrant and garlic is light brown; mix with shredded meat; set aside.

Heat beef broth and water in a large saucepan. Add bok choy, mushrooms, and drained, soaked mung bean noodles; cook about 3-4 minutes until noodles are just soft and bok choy is cooked. Add marinated meat and scallions to soup and heat through. Divide among bowls; serve with extra Korean red pepper flakes for spicy food lovers. If beef broth is unsalted, serve with fish sauce or soy sauce on the side for drizzling.

Per serving: 314 calories, 8 g fat (5 g sat), 22 g protein, 18 g carb, 677 mg sodium, 1 g sugars, 1 g fiber

NOOM CROCKPOT BEEF VEGETABLE SOUP

Ingredients:

1 Tbsp extra virgin olive oil

1 lb boneless chuck roast or beef stew meat — cut into 1-inch cubes

2 tsp kosher salt — divided

¼ tsp black pepper

3-4 c. low sodium beef broth — divided

1 small yellow onion — diced

2 cloves garlic — minced (about 2 tsp)

4 large carrots — peeled and finely chopped

2 Yukon gold potatoes — peeled and diced

2 parsnips — peeled and diced

2 ribs celery — diced

1 14.5-ounce can diced tomatoes

1 can tomato sauce (8 ounces)

3 Tbsp tomato paste

1 Tbsp Worcestershire sauce

1 tsp dried oregano

½ tsp smoked paprika

½ tsp granulated sugar

1 c. peas — fresh or frozen (no need to thaw)

Chopped fresh parsley — optional for serving

Directions:

In a large skillet, heat the oil over medium high. Add the beef and sprinkle with 1 teaspoon salt and pepper. Brown the beef on all sides, disturbing it as little as possible on each side so that it develops nice coloring. Once the beef is lightly browned (it won't be all the way cooked through), remove it to a 6-quart slow cooker.

To the pan, add the onion. Cook and stir until the onion is beginning to soften, about 3 minutes. Stir in the garlic and let cook 30 seconds. Splash in about 1/2 cup the beef broth and scrape up any browned bits that have stuck to the bottom (this is flavor!). Let the broth reduce for 2 minutes, then transfer the entire mixture to the slow cooker.

To the slow cooker, add the carrots, potatoes, parsnips, celery, diced tomatoes in their juices, tomato sauce, tomato paste, Worcestershire, oregano, paprika, sugar, 2 1/2 cups beef broth, and remaining 1 teaspoon salt.

Cover and cook on low for 8 hours, until the beef and vegetables are tender. Stir in the peas, just until warmed through. If the soup is thicker than you would like, add the remaining 1 cup beef broth until you reach your desired consistency. Serve hot, sprinkled with fresh parsley.

Per serving: 283 calories, 7 g fat (2 g sat), 24 g protein, 33 g carb, 11 g sugars, 8 g fiber

Mediterranean Shrimp

Ingredients:

1 lb large shrimp — 40 to 50 per pound peeled, deveined shrimp, tails on or off (fresh or frozen and thawed)

¾ tsp kosher salt — divided

½ tsp ground black pepper — divided

2 Tbsp extra virgin olive oil

1 small red onion — chopped

2 cloves garlic — minced (about 2 teaspoons)

1 14.5-oz can fire roasted diced tomatoes in their juices

1 tsp dried oregano

¼ tsp red pepper flakes

1 tsp honey

1 tsp red wine vinegar

1 14-oz can artichoke hearts — drained and quartered

½ c. pitted Kalamata olives

¾ c. crumbled feta cheese

2 Tbsp chopped fresh parsley

2 Tbsp fresh lemon juice — from about ½ medium lemon

For serving: rice — whole wheat couscous, crusty bread, pasta (optional)

Directions:

Place a rack in the center of your oven and preheat the oven to 400 degrees F. Pat the shrimp dry, place in a mixing bowl, and sprinkle with ½ teaspoon salt and ¼ teaspoon black pepper. Toss to coat, then set aside.

In a large, ovenproof skillet over medium heat, heat the olive oil. Add onion and sprinkle with the remaining ¼ teaspoon salt and ¼ teaspoon black pepper. Cook, stirring occasionally, until softened, about 5 minutes. Reduce the heat as needed so that the onion softens but does not brown. Add the garlic and cook just until fragrant, about 30 seconds.

Add the tomatoes, oregano, and red pepper flakes. Reduce the heat to medium-low and let gently simmer for 10 minutes. Stir in the red wine vinegar and honey. Remove from the heat.

Scatter the artichokes and olives over the top, then arrange the shrimp on top in a single layer. Sprinkle with the feta.

Bake for 10 to 12 minutes, until the tomatoes are bubbling, cheese has browned slightly, and the shrimp are cooked through. Squeeze the lemon juice over the top and sprinkle with parsley. Enjoy hot.

Per serving: 445 calories, 24 g fat (8 g sat), 38 g protein, 17 g carb, 9 g sugars, 3 g fiber

MEXICAN STUFFED PEPPERS

Ingredients:

4 large bell peppers

2 tsp extra virgin olive oil

1 lb ground chicken — or turkey (I used chicken)

1 tsp ground chili powder

1 tsp ground cumin

1 tsp garlic powder

½ tsp kosher salt

¼ tsp black pepper

1 can fire-roasted diced tomatoes — with juices, 14 ounces

1 ½ c. cooked brown rice — quinoa or cauliflower rice

1 ¼ c. shredded cheese — Monterey Jack, pepper jack, cheddar, or similar cheese, divided

Directions:

Preheat your oven to 375 degrees F. Lightly coat a 9x13-inch baking dish with nonstick spray. Slice the bell peppers in half from top to bottom. Remove the seeds and membranes, then arrange cut side up in the prepared baking dish.

Heat the olive oil in a large, nonstick skillet over medium high heat. Add the chicken, chili powder, cumin, garlic powder, salt, and pepper. Cook, breaking apart the meat, until the chicken is browned and cooked through, about 4 minutes. Drain off any excess liquid, then pour in the can of diced tomatoes and their juices. Let simmer for 1 minute.

Remove the pan from the heat. Stir in the rice and ¾ cup of the shredded cheese. Mound the filling inside of the peppers, then top with the remaining cheese.

Pour a bit of water into the pan with the peppers—just enough to barely cover the bottom of the pan. Bake uncovered for 25 to 35 minutes, until the peppers are tender and the cheese is melted. Top with any of your favorite fixings, and enjoy hot.

Per serving: 438 calories, 20 g fat (8 g sat), 32 g protein, 32 g carb, 8 g sugars, 5 g fiber

Zucchini Pizza Boats

Ingredients:

4 medium zucchini

¼ tsp kosher salt

1 c. pizza sauce — or similar prepared marinara sauce

1 ¼ c. shredded mozzarella cheese — or a blend of shredded mozzarella and provolone

1 tsp Italian seasoning

¼ - ½ tsp crushed red pepper flakes — optional

¼ c. mini pepperoni — or mini turkey pepperoni or regular-size pepperoni, sliced into quarters

2 tsp freshly ground Parmesan

2 tsp chopped fresh basil, thyme, or other fresh herbs

Directions:

Place a rack in the center of your oven. Preheat the oven to 375 degrees F. Lightly coat a rimmed baking sheet or 9x13-inch baking dish with nonstick spray.

Halve each zucchini lengthwise. With a small spoon or melon baller, gently scrape out the center zucchini flesh and pulp, leaving a border of about 1/3 inch on all sides. Arrange the zucchini shells on the baking sheet. Sprinkle the insides of the zucchini with salt.

Spoon the pizza sauce into each shell, dividing it evenly. You may need a little more or less, depending upon the size of your zucchini. Put a generous amount, but don't feel like you need to fill it all the way to the very top.

Sprinkle the mozzarella over the top, then evenly sprinkle with Italian seasoning and red pepper flakes (if using). Scatter on the pepperoni and any other desired toppings. Last, sprinkle with Parmesan.

Bake for 15 to 20 minutes, until the cheese is hot and bubbly and the zucchini is tender. If desired, switch the oven to broil and cook the zucchini for 2 to 3 additional minutes, until the cheese is lightly browned. Remove from the oven and sprinkle with chopped fresh basil. Serve immediately.

Per serving: 100 calories, 6 g fat (3 g sat), 7 g protein, 5 g carb, 4 g sugars, 2 g fiber

Creamy Gluten-Free Tomato Pasta

Ingredients:

3 Tbsp olive oil (divided)

½ c. diced white onion

1 tsp minced garlic

10 oz gluten free pasta

8 oz canned Italian stewed tomatoes (drained)

¼ c. paleo mayo

1 egg yolk

¼ tsp each kosher salt and black pepper

Optional ½ tsp crushed red pepper flakes

Fresh basil and cracked pepper

Directions:

In a small pan, sauté onions and garlic in 1 tbsp olive until fragrant, about 2 minutes. Once they are almost cooked, set aside.

In a large pot, cook your gluten free pasta according to directions.

Drain, rinse the pasta, and place pasta back into pot. Keep on low heat.

Mix in the remaining 2 tbsp olive oil and mix well. Mix gently.

In a separate bowl, whisk together the mayo and egg yolk.

Add this mix to your pot with the pasta, coating until creamy. Gently mix in the sauteed onion/garlic.

Toss the pasta with the tomatoes, kosher salt and pepper.

Stir gently over low to medium low heat until creamy and combined.

If using a cooked protein, add it in here.

Plate pasta into bowls. Garnish with fresh basil and cracked pepper.

Per serving: 353 calories, 17.1 g fat (2.7 g sat), 9.2 g protein, 42.2 g carb, 186 mg sodium, 4.8 g sugars, 3.7 g fiber

HONEY MUSTARD CHICKEN WITH BRUSSEL SPROUTS

Ingredients:

Nonstick cooking spray

1/4 c. plus 2 tablespoons extra-virgin olive oil

2 Tbsp fresh lemon juice (1 lemon)

1 Tbsp Dijon mustard

1 Tbsp whole-grain mustard

1 Tbsp honey

3 garlic cloves, minced

Kosher salt and freshly ground black pepper

2 lb bone-in, skin-on chicken thighs (4 medium thighs)

1 1/2 lb Brussels sprouts, halved

1/4 large red onion, sliced

Directions:

Preheat the oven to 425°F. Grease a large baking sheet with nonstick cooking spray and set aside.

In a medium bowl, whisk together the 1/4 cup olive oil, 1 tablespoon of the lemon juice, the Dijon mustard, whole-grain mustard, honey, and garlic. Season with salt and pepper to taste.

Use tongs to dip the chicken thighs in the sauce, coating both sides. Place the thighs on the prepared baking sheet. Discard any remaining sauce.

In a medium bowl, combine the Brussels sprouts and red onion. Drizzle with the remaining 2 tablespoons olive oil and 1 tablespoon lemon juice and toss until well coated. Arrange the sprouts around the chicken on the baking sheet, making sure they aren't overlapping. Season with salt and pepper.

Roast for 30 to 35 minutes, until the chicken is golden brown and has an internal temperature of 165°F and the Brussels sprouts are crispy. Serve hot.

Per serving: 360 calories, 20.1 g fat (3.6 g sat), 30.8 g protein, 14.5 g carb, 350.8 mg sodium, 6.8 g sugars, 3.7 g fiber

Chinese Cauliflower Fried Rice Casserole

Ingredients:

Sesame oil for the pan

Optional 5 oz diced meat (pork or chicken)

1 Tbsp grated ginger

1 small shallot, chopped

2 tsp garlic, minced

1 lb stir fry vegetables

Handful of mung bean sprouts, optional

¼ c. gluten free Szechuan sauce or other gluten-free sauce of choice

3 c. cauliflower rice or broccoli rice (about 1 small to medium head of cauliflower)

2 Tbsp beef broth (you can skip if your veggies are less starchy. The broth just gives the casserole more flavor.)

6 eggs (2 in stir fry and 4 on top, soft baked)

Directions:

Preheat oven to 350 F.

Add 1-2 Tbsp sesame oil to a wok or large pan and heat to medium high. If you are wanting to add meat, do so here. Simply stir fry until browned and mostly cooked (in sesame oil), then remove meat and set aside. If you are making the vegetarian option, skip the browning and go straight to adding your shallot, ginger, and garlic to the wok/pan and stir fry ingredients until fragrant – about 2 minutes.

Next add all of your stir fry veggies and sauce. Stir fry for 2-3 minutes again until well coated.

Mix in your cauliflower rice, broth, and 2 eggs. The 2 eggs can be added to the stir fry whole, or whisked then added. Either works!

Stir fry for an additional 3-4 minutes to create a fried cauliflower rice. All in all, the stir frying should not take longer than 10 minutes.

Transfer wok/pan ingredients to an 8 x 11 casserole dish or baking dish.

Crack 4 eggs on top of the casserole, spacing them out evenly. Cover with foil, and place in oven at 350F for 15-20 minutes or until eggs are set. For runny eggs, remove casserole from oven after 12-15 minutes of baking and slice the yolk in the middle to create a runny egg (similar to pictures in blog).

Return casserole to the oven for an additional 3-5 minutes.

Cool before freezing, or serve immediately.

Garnish with green onion, cilantro, sesame seeds and optional red pepper flakes.

Per serving: 165 calories, 8.8 g fat (2.4 g sat), 11 g protein, 11.8 g carb, 387.4 mg sodium, 6.2 g sugars, 2.8 g fiber

MEXICAN SALAD WITH CHIPOTLE SHRIMP

Ingredients:

2 lb raw jumbo shrimp, peeled and cleaned (tail on or off)

8 c. chopped kale

4 ears corn on the cob, shucked

15 oz can black beans, drained

1 pint grape or cherry tomatoes, halved

1 whole ripe avocado, peeled and chopped

2-3 whole chipotle peppers in adobo sauce

7 Tbsp fresh lime juice, divided

¼ c. olive oil

¼ c. mayonnaise

2 Tbsp honey

3 cloves garlic

½ tsp salt

Directions:

Preheat the grill to medium heat. To a blender jar, add the chipotle peppers, 4 tablespoons of lime juice, olive oil, garlic, and salt. Cover and puree until smooth.

Measure out 3 tablespoons of the chipotle puree and save it for the dressing. In a medium bowl, mix the shrimp and the remaining marinade, until well coated.

In a separate small bowl, mix the 3 tablespoons of chipotle puree, 3 tablespoons lime juice, mayonnaise, and honey. Whisk until smooth. Then taste, and salt and pepper as needed.

Prep all the veggies. Set out a large salad bowl. Add the kale. Then toss it with the dressing until well coated. (I like to massage the dressing into the kale by hand.) Then add in the black beans, tomatoes, and avocado.

Place the shrimp and corn cobs on the grills. *If your shrimp are small they will fall through the grates. Either use a grill basket, or place them on a piece of foil. Grill the shrimp for 3-5 minutes until pink. Grill the corn for 8-10 minutes rotating every 2 minutes.

Once the corn is cool enough to handle, cut it off the cobs and add it to the salad. Then toss in the shrimp and serve.

Per serving: 372 calories, 15 g fat (2 g sat), 31 g protein, 31 g carb, 1314 mg sodium, 9 g sugars, 5 g fiber

Chicken Sausage Apple Squash Sheet Pan Dinner

Ingredients:

1 Tbsp olive oil

1 small butternut squash

1 large crisp apple

1 sweet onion

4 chicken sausages

½ Tbsp ground allspice

Salt and pepper

Directions:

Preheat the oven to 425 degrees F. Cut the butternut squash in half, lengthwise. Cut off the circular orb sections (the end with the seedpod) and save for future use.

Peel the long sections of the butternut squash, then slice them into thin wedges. Core the apple and slice into wedges, unpeeled. Then peel and slice the onion into wedges.

Pile the butternut squash, apples, and onions on a large rimmed 18x13-inch "half sheet" baking pan. Drizzle olive oil over the top and toss to coat. Then spread the squash, apples, and onions out into a single layer. Sprinkle with allspice, salt, and pepper.

Roast in the oven for 15 minutes. Meanwhile, cut the chicken sausages on the bias, into 1/2-inch slices.

Flip the veggies, and spread them back out. Make room on the baking sheet to add the sausages. Place the sheet back in the oven for 10-15 minutes, until the sausages are sizzling. Serve warm!

Per serving: 336 calories, 15 g fat (3 g sat), 15 g protein, 38 g carb, 884 mg sodium, 14 g sugars, 5 g fiber

Confetti Quinoa Stuffed Chicken

Ingredients:

4 boneless skinless chicken breasts

¾ c. quinoa, any color

1 ½ c. chicken broth

1 Tbsp coconut oil

¾ c. diced bell pepper (I used red and yellow)

½ c. diced red onion

2 cloves garlic, minced

1 serrano pepper, seeded and diced

? c. shaved unsweetened coconut (coconut chips)

¼ c. chipped cilantro

1 lime, zest and 1 tablespoon juice

1 tsp ground cumin

1 tsp chili powder

1 tsp salt

Directions:

Preheat the oven to 375 degrees F. Line a rimmed baking sheet with parchment paper. Place the coconut oil in a medium sauce pot and set over medium-high heat. Once melted, add the diced bell pepper, red onion, garlic, and serrano pepper. Sauté for 1-2 minutes to soften just a little. Then pour the vegetables into a bowl. They should still be bright in color.

Place the quinoa in the empty sauce pot. Turn the heat up to high and add the broth and 1/2 teaspoon salt. Cover the pot and bring to a boil. Cook for 15 minutes, or until the broth has absorbed and there are vent holes in the surface of the quinoa. Remove from heat and let the quinoa steam for another 5 minutes.

Meanwhile, use a boning knife to cut a slit in each chicken breast along one long side. Cut through the center of the chicken, with the knife parallel to the cutting board, leaving the opposite side attached. You're trying to create a deep pocket in each breast, with a 1/2-inch border around the three attached sides. (See post images for clarification.) Cut evenly, as to not leave thick uncut sections that won't cook through in the oven. Then sprinkle each breast on all sides with cumin, chili powder, and salt.

Once the quinoa is fluffy, stir in the sautéed vegetables, shaved coconut, cilantro, lime zest, and lime juice. Taste, and salt as needed. Stuff the confetti quinoa into the cavity of each chicken breast. Stand the chicken breasts up on the baking sheet, like open envelopes, with the quinoa on top.

Bake for 20 minutes. Serve warm.

Per serving: 355 calories, 13 g fat (8 g sat), 30 g protein, 28 g carb, 1051 mg sodium, 2 g sugars, 4 g fiber

ONE-POT CHICKEN SOUP WITH WHITE BEANS & KALE

Ingredients:

1 strip uncured bacon, chopped

1 Tbsp avocado oil (if using bacon, omit oil)

1 c. diced white or yellow onion

4 cloves garlic, minced

8 c. broth (chicken broth or vegetable broth)

1 15-oz can white beans, slightly drained

2 c. shredded chicken

Sea salt and black pepper to taste

3 c. loosely packed chopped kale (or other sturdy green)

Directions:

Heat a large pot or Dutch oven over medium heat. Once hot, add bacon (optional) or oil. Let heat for 1 minute, stirring occasionally. Then add onion.

Sauté for 4-5 minutes, stirring occasionally, or until onion is translucent and fragrant. Then add garlic and sauté 2-3 minutes more, being careful not to burn.

Next add broth, slightly drained white beans, and chicken and bring to a simmer. Cook for 10 minutes to meld the flavors. Then taste and season with salt and pepper to taste. In the last few minutes of cooking, add the kale, cover, and cook until wilted.

Serve hot. Store cooled leftovers covered in the fridge up to 3-4 days, or in the freezer up to 1 month. Reheat in the microwave or on the stovetop until hot.

Per serving: 201 calories, 6.9 g fat (1.6 g sat), 15.8 g protein, 19.5 g carb, 689 mg sodium, 2.3 g sugars, 15.8 g fiber

Balsamic-Marinated Portobello Pizzas

Ingredients:

4 large portobello mushrooms (stems removed, wiped clean)

¼ c. balsamic vinegar

2 Tbsp avocado or olive oil

1 pinch salt and pepper (or red pepper flake)

1 medium red bell pepper (cut into bite-size pieces)

1 small red onion (thinly sliced wedges or diced)

1 head garlic (cloves separated and peeled)

2 Tbsp avocado or olive oil

1 healthy pinch sea salt and black pepper (or red pepper flake)

2 Tbsp fresh herbs (such as rosemary or oregano // optional)

¾ c. pizza sauce

½ c. sun-dried tomatoes (if large, chop into smaller pieces // we prefer Trader Joe's brand)

? c. soft vegan cheese, divided

Directions:

Preheat oven to 400 degrees F (204 C) and line a large baking sheet with parchment paper. Set aside.

Add portobello mushrooms (stem side up) to a shallow dish or large freezer bag. Add the balsamic vinegar, oil, salt and pepper (or red pepper flake). Use a pastry brush to brush on all sides (or shake bag to coat). Marinate on one side for 5 minutes, then the other side for 5 minutes.

In the meantime, add vegetables and garlic to baking sheet, toss with oil, salt and pepper, and fresh herbs (optional) and bake for 20-25 minutes or until golden brown and fragrant, tossing once near the halfway point to ensure even baking. Set aside but keep oven at 400 F (204 C).

If serving with balsamic reduction (see notes) and/or soft nut cheese (see links above), prepare at this time.

Heat a large skillet over medium heat (you could also use a grill for this step). Add mushrooms to the pan, leaving any leftover oil-and-vinegar marinade behind. Cook on each side for about 4-5 minutes, or until caramelized and softened. If your mushrooms are extra thick, covering with a lid can be helpful to encourage even cooking all the way through. Brush on any remaining marinade while cooking to infuse more flavor.

Once mushrooms and vegetables are cooked, assemble pizzas. Place mushrooms on a parchment-lined baking sheet or baking pan and add toppings, starting with pizza sauce, then roasted veggies, roasted garlic, and soft vegan cheese. You can also add vegan parmesan cheese or red pepper flake at this point (optional).

Bake for about 15-20 minutes or until hot. The soft vegan cheese will be slightly golden brown on top. Remove from oven and enjoy as is, or garnish with sun-dried tomatoes, fresh basil, balsamic drizzle, red pepper flake, and extra vegan parmesan (all optional).

Per serving: 301 calories, 21.6 g fat (2.8 g sat), 5.5 g protein, 22.5 g carb, 179 mg sodium, 12.1 g sugars, 4.6 g fiber

CHICKEN AND ZUCCHINI STIR FRY

Ingredients:

¼ c. low sodium soy sauce or use gluten-free soy sauce

1 c. chicken broth

1 Tbsp cornstarch

2 Tbsp mirin

1 Tbsp sugar

2 tsp sesame oil

1 tsp canola oil divided

1 Tbsp minced garlic

1 Tbsp minced ginger

1 lb chicken breast, sliced very thinly

2 c. zucchini, cut ¼ inch thick half moons (from 1 large zucchini)

Sesame seeds and scallion for garnish, if desired

Directions:

In a large bowl add the soy sauce, chicken broth, cornstarch, mirin, sugar, and sesame oil and whisk until everything is completely dissolved.

In a large skillet add one teaspoon canola oil on medium high heat and cook half the chicken until just cooked through, about 2-3 minutes on each side. Set aside on a plate.

Repeat with the second half of the chicken and an additional teaspoon of oil. Remove the chicken to the plate.

Add in the remaining 1 teaspoon oil, garlic and ginger and cook for 30-45 seconds until very fragrant but not browned.

Stir the garlic and ginger well and add in the sauce, whisking well. Cook the sauce 1 minute, then add in the zucchini and cook for 2 minutes more, until thickened and the zucchini is tender crisp. Remove from heat, add in the chicken and stir well to coat. Garnish with sesame seeds and scallions if desired.

Per serving: 242 calories, 6.5 g fat (1 g sat), 28 g protein, 17 g carb, 799 mg sodium, 8 g sugars, 1.5 g fiber

Broiled Tilapia with Thai Coconut Curry Sauce

Ingredients:

1 tsp dark sesame oil, divided

1 Tbsp minced peeled fresh ginger

4 garlic cloves, minced

1 c. finely chopped red bell pepper

1 c. chopped scallions

1 tsp curry powder

2 tsp red curry paste

½ tsp ground cumin

4 tsp low-sodium soy sauce, use tamari for gluten-free

1 Tbsp brown sugar

2 tsp Asian fish sauce

1 14-oz can light coconut milk

¼ c. chopped fresh cilantro

6 6-oz tilapia fillets

Salt

Directions:

Preheat broiler.

Heat ½ teaspoon oil in a large nonstick skillet over medium heat. Add the ginger, garlic, pepper and scallions; cook 1 minute. Stir in curry powder, curry paste, and cumin; cook 1 minute.

Add soy sauce, sugar, Asian fish sauce, and coconut milk; bring to a simmer (do not boil). Remove from heat; stir in cilantro or basil if using.

Brush fish with ½ teaspoon oil; sprinkle with ¼ teaspoon salt. Place fish on a baking sheet coated with cooking spray.

Broil 7 minutes or until fish flakes easily when tested with a fork.

Serve fish with sauce, rice, and lime wedges.

Per serving: 225 calories, 7 g fat (0 g sat), 35.5 g protein, 5.5 g carb, 1.1 g fiber

Sheet Pan Turkey Meatloaf and Broccoli

Ingredients:

1.3 lb (20 oz) 93% ground turkey

? c. quick cooking oatmeal, or gf oats

6 Tbsp ketchup, divided

? c. minced onion

1 large egg

½ tsp dried or fresh thyme leaves

1 tsp kosher salt

2 tsp Worcesterchire sauce, divided

1 large bunch broccoli, (1 ½ pounds) cut into florets

2 Tbsp olive oil

¾ tsp kosher salt

Directions:

Preheat the oven to 425F. Line a 13x9-inch sheet pan with Reynolds Wrap Non-Stick Foil, dull side facing up towards food.

In a medium bowl toss broccoli with oil and season with ½ teaspoon salt and spread out on the sheet pan in a single layer on one side.

In a medium bowl combine ground turkey, oatmeal, ¼ cup ketchup, onion, egg, ¾ teaspoon salt, 1 teaspoon Worcesterchire sauce and thyme, mix well.

Divide mixture into 4 equal portions. Shape each portion into a

4 x 3-inch free form loaf on the other side of the sheet pan.

In a small bowl mix remaining 2 tablespoons ketchup with remaining teaspoon of Worcestershire sauce and brush onto loaves.

Bake 30 minutes in the center of the oven, turning the broccoli halfway, until meat is cooked through in the center and the broccoli is slightly charred.

Per serving: 335 calories, 13 g fat (4 g sat), 35 g protein, 22.5 g carb, 933 mg sodium, 4 g sugars, 6g fiber

NOOM SPICY TUNA POKE BOWLS

Ingredients:

½ lb sushi grade tuna, cut into 1/2-inch cubes

¼ c. sliced scallions

2 Tbsp reduced sodium soy sauce or gluten-free tamari

1 tsp sesame oil

½ tsp sriracha

2 Tbsp light mayonnaise

2 tsp sriracha sauce

1 c. cooked short grain brown rice or sushi white rice

1 c. cucumbers, (from 2 Persian) peeled and diced ½-inch cubes

½ medium Hass avocado, (3 ounces) sliced

2 scallions, sliced for garnish

1 tsp black sesame seeds

Reduced sodium soy or gluten-free tamari, for serving (optional)

Sriracha, for serving (optional)

Directions:

In a small bowl combine the mayonnaise and sriracha, thin with a little water to drizzle.

In a medium bowl, combine tuna with scallions, soy sauce, sesame oil and sriracha. Gently toss to combine and set aside while you prepare the bowls.

In 2 bowls, layer 1/2 the rice, 1/2 the tuna, avocado, cucumber and scallions.

Drizzle with spicy mayo and sesame seeds and serve with extra soy sauce on the side, if desired.

Per serving: 397 calories, 14.5 g fat (2 g sat), 32.5 g protein, 33.5 g carb, 864.5 mg sodium, 3 g sugars, 6 g fiber

Egg Roll in a Bowl

Ingredients:

1 lb ground chicken or turkey

2 tsp fresh ginger, grated or minced

¼ c. chopped yellow onion

2 cloves garlic, minced

2 tsp sesame oil

1 12-oz package coleslaw or broccoli slaw mix

3 Tbsp coconut aminos (or low-sodium tamari or soy sauce)

1 tsp sambal oelek paste

2 green onions, chopped

Sriracha, for serving (optional)

Sesame seeds and cilantro, for garnish (optional)

Directions:

Brown ground chicken or turkey in a large skillet. Break meat into smaller pieces as it cooks using a wooden spoon or spatula. Cook for about 6-8 minutes or until the meat is no longer pink. Remove from heat.

In the same skillet over medium heat, add sesame oil. Once hot, add onion, garlic and ginger and cook until fragrant, about 3-5 minutes. Add coleslaw mix (shredded cabbage and carrots) into the skillet. Toss and add coconut aminos and sambal oelek paste. Cook for another 3-5 minutes or until cabbage is tender.

Portion into bowls and top each with green onions and a drizzle of sriracha, sesame seeds and cilantro (if using).

Per serving: 325 calories, 15 g fat (3 g sat), 32 g protein, 14 g carb, 393 mg sodium, 8 g sugars, 3 g fiber

BLACKENED CHICKEN COBB SALAD

Ingredients:

¾ tsp paprika

¾ tsp chili powder

¾ tsp garlic powder

½ tsp sea salt

¼ tsp pepper

Pinch of cayenne pepper

1 Tbsp olive oil (if needed)

1 lb boneless skinless chicken breasts (3–4 pieces)

12 c. baby spinach or chopped romaine

4 large eggs, hard-boiled, peeled and sliced

1 c. grape tomatoes, halved

1 large cucumber, sliced

1 c. baby bella mushrooms, sautéed

½ c. red onion, chopped

6 slices cooked turkey bacon, crumbled

½ c. crumbled blue cheese (optional)

1–2 avocados, sliced

Ingredients for the red wine vinaigrette:

? c. red wine vinegar

1 Tbsp Dijon mustard

1 tsp maple syrup or honey

¾ tsp sea salt

½ tsp black pepper

½ c. extra virgin olive oil

Directions:

Take chicken out of the package and pat dry with paper towels. Add spices — paprika, garlic powder, chili powder, sea salt, black pepper and cayenne pepper — in a small bowl. Coat each chicken breast with spice mixture.

To cook the chicken, you can either grill it on an indoor or outdoor grill or sear it on the stovetop. To sear: add 1 Tablespoon olive oil to a large skillet over medium heat. Place chicken breasts in hot oil. Cook chicken about 6–7 minutes on each side, or until juices run clear. Remove chicken from skillet and let sit for 5 minutes to cool before slicing for the salad. This step can be done a day in advance.

While the chicken cooks, make the dressing by whisking together all the ingredients in a small bowl or glass jar.

Divide the spinach or romaine among 4 plates (or containers if you're making this for meal prep). Arrange equal portions of blackened chicken, hard-boiled egg, tomatoes, cucumber, mushrooms, red onion, avocado, bacon and blue cheese on top of the greens.

Just before serving, top salad with 1–2 Tablespoons of the red wine vinaigrette dressing or your favorite dressing.

Per serving: 475 calories, 25 g fat, 46 g protein, 17 g carb, 5 g sugars, 9 g fiber

Asian Chicken Lettuce Wraps

Ingredients:

3 Tbsp hoisin sauce

2 Tbsp low-sodium tamari (or soy sauce)

2 Tbsp rice wine vinegar

1 Tbsp Sriracha

1 tsp sesame oil

1 Tbsp avocado or olive oil

1 medium onion, diced

2 cloves garlic, minced

1 Tbsp freshly grated ginger

1 lb ground chicken

½ c. water chestnuts, drained and sliced

Sea salt and black pepper, to taste

Butter, Bibb or Iceberg lettuce (leaves separated), for serving

2 green onions, thinly sliced, for serving

¼ c. crushed peanuts, for serving

Ingredients for the peanut sauce:

¼ c. peanut butter

2 Tbsp low sodium tamari (or soy sauce)

2 Tbsp maple syrup

1 clove garlic

1 tsp Sriracha

Water

Directions:

Whisk together hoisin sauce, soy sauce, rice wine vinegar, Sriracha and sesame oil in a small bowl. Set aside.

In a large skillet over medium-high heat, heat oil. Add onions and cook until soft, 5 minutes, then stir in garlic and ginger and cook until fragrant, 1 minute more. Add ground chicken and cook until opaque and mostly cooked through, breaking up meat with a wooden spoon.

Pour in sauce and cook 1 to 2 minutes more, until sauce reduces slightly and chicken is cooked through completely. Turn off heat and stir in water chestnuts. Taste mixture and season with salt and pepper, if needed.

Make peanut sauce by whisking together all ingredients in a small bowl. For a thinner sauce, add water 1 Tablespoon at a time to create the desired consistency.

Serve chicken mixture with lettuce leaves and spoon about 1/4 cup into center of each leaf. Top with crushed peanuts and green onions. Serve with peanut sauce.

Per serving: 471 calories, 29 g fat, 28 g protein, 28 g carb, 908 mg sodium, 17 g sugars, 3 g fiber

. CHIPOTLE CHICKEN TOSTADAS WITH PINEAPPLE SALSA

Ingredients:

1 Tbsp avocado oil (or olive oil)

2 lb ground chicken

2 tsp chipotle chili powder

Freshly ground salt and pepper

¼ c. low-sodium chicken broth

1 Tbsp tomato paste

6 (8-inch) grain-free tortillas

2 avocados, mashed

½ c. shredded purple cabbage

¼ c. chopped fresh cilantro leaves

Ingredients for the pineapple salsa:

2 c. small diced fresh pineapple

¼ c. finely diced red onion

1 Tbsp finely diced jalapeño

2 Tbsp fresh lime juice (from 1 lime)

1 garlic clove, minced

1 Tbsp finely chopped fresh cilantro leaves

1 tsp avocado oil (or olive oil)

Pinch of salt

Directions:

Preheat the oven to 350 degrees F and line a baking sheet with parchment paper.

Make the pineapple salsa: in a medium bowl, toss together the pineapple, onion, jalapeño, lime juice, garlic, cilantro, avocado oil and salt. Refrigerate until ready to serve, up to 5 days.

Make the chicken: in a large skillet, heat the avocado oil over medium-high heat. Add the ground chicken, chipotle chili powder, salt and pepper.

Cook the chicken, breaking up the meat with the back of a spoon until it is brown, about 7 minutes. Drain off any excess fat from the pan, if necessary.

Reduce the heat to medium and add the chicken broth and tomato paste and stir to combine. Continue to cook for about 2 more minutes.

Remove from heat and cover to keep warm until ready to serve.

To assemble: place the tortillas in a single layer on the prepared baking sheet. Lightly spray the tops of tortillas with nonstick cooking spray. Bake for 8 to 10 minutes, or until golden brown and crisp.

Carefully spread the mashed avocado on top of each crisp tortilla. Sprinkle with the shredded cabbage and a big scoop of chipotle chicken. Top with the pineapple salsa and a sprinkle of cilantro.

Per serving: 462 calories, 26.7 g fat (6.3 g sat), 31.8 g protein, 26.8 g carb, 7.1 g sugars, 7 g fiber

CREAMY CHIPOTLE SWEET POTATO PENNE PASTA

Ingredients:

3 c. of brown rice and quinoa penne

1/2 Tbsp olive oil

1 c. sliced baby bella mushrooms

1/4 tsp garlic powder

Freshly ground pepper and salt, to taste

Ingredients for the sauce:

½ c. whole cashews, soaked for 2 hours and drained

1 small roasted sweet potato, skin removed

? c. water

2 cloves garlic

1 Pueblo Lindo Chiles Chipotle Pepper (can add one more if you like extra spice!)

? tsp nutmeg

½ tsp salt, plus more to taste

Freshly ground pepper

Directions:

Make sure you soak the cashews in 4 cups of water for at least 2 hours, otherwise you can place them large bowl, then add 4 cups boiling water and let the cashews soak in the hot water for approximately 45 minutes to speed up the process.

Once ready to make the pasta sauce: add drained cashews, roasted sweet potato, water, garlic, chipotle chile pepper, nutmeg, salt and pepper to a high powered blender. Blend until a thick sauce comes together, adding a tablespoon or two more of water, if necessary to help blend. Taste and adjust seasonings as necessary. Set aside for later.

Boil the pasta according to the directions on the package. Drain pasta, then transfer back to pot.

While the pasta is boiling, sauté your mushrooms: add olive oil to a skillet and place over medium heat. Add mushrooms and then season with garlic powder, salt and pepper; sauté for 3-5 minutes until mushrooms are cooked and look nice and juicy.

Stir sweet potato sauce into the cooked pasta. Add mushrooms and stir again. Garnish with sage or parsley, whatever you prefer. Serves 4.

Per serving: 456 calories, 12.2 g fat (1.8 g sat), 11.4 g protein, 76.9 g carb, 2.8 g sugars, 4.9 g fiber

Spinach Garlic Parmesan Orzo with Crispy Bacon

Ingredients:

8 slices bacon

10 oz uncooked orzo pasta (about 1 2/3 c. uncooked orzo)

½ c. reserved pasta water, after pasta is done boiling

1 Tbsp butter

3 cloves garlic, finely minced

½ c. shredded carrots (or carrots cut into matchsticks)

? c. frozen or fresh sweet corn

1 red bell pepper, cut into chunks

1 (5-oz) package organic spinach

½ c. freshly grated parmesan cheese

½ tsp garlic powder

½ tsp red chili pepper flakes, plus more if desired

Freshly ground salt and pepper

Directions:

Add bacon to a large skillet or pan and place over medium heat, cook bacon on both sides until crispy and golden brown. If the pan starts to smoke at any point, simply lower the heat. I always cook my bacon on medium low heat. Once bacon is done, blot with a paper towel to absorb excess grease, then chop into bite sized pieces and set aside.

While the bacon is cooking, place a large pot of water over high heat and add in a generous amount of salt. Once water boils, stir in the orzo and cook until al dente about 7-9 minutes. Once orzo is done cooking, drain pasta and set aside in the colander. Make sure to reserve ½ cup of the pasta water.

Next add 1 tablespoon butter to the same pot you cooked the

pasta in and place over medium heat. Once butter is melted, add in minced garlic, carrot, corn, red bell pepper and saute for 2 minutes.

Next add in spinach; cooking until the spinach wilts, about 2 minutes. Add the cooked orzo back into the pot and turn the heat to low. Stir in the reserved pasta water, parmesan, garlic powder and red chili pepper flakes.

Finally, stir in bacon crumbles. Add salt and pepper to taste. I like to add A LOT of black pepper into this dish -- it just gives it a really nice flavor! If you think it needs a little extra parmesan cheese, feel free to stir in ¼ cup more. Enjoy. Serves 4.

Per serving: 436 calories, 13.3 g fat (6.2 g sat), 20.2 g protein, 62.7 g carb, 2.6 g sugars, 4.5 g fiber

ROSEMARY CITRUS ONE PAN BAKED SALMON

Ingredients:

1/3 cup olive oil

Pinch of ground pepper

2 Tbsp fresh orange juice

2 Tbsp fresh rosemary, plus 1-2 extra sprigs to garnish

1 Tbsp Lemon juice

1/2 tsp garlic minced

1/4 tsp of grated dried orange peel (divided)

Kosher salt or fine sea salt to taste

1 bunch thin asparagus (trimmed) (Or other vegetable of choice)

Olive oil or melted butter to drizzle

10–12 ounces sockeye salmon (whole fillet or around 3 fillets)

Thinly sliced Orange (5-6)

Optional 1/4 tsp lemon pepper

Additional Salt/pepper to taste – after baking

Direction

Preheat oven to 400 degrees F.

Whisk together orange juice, lemon, 2 Tbsp rosemary, 1/4 to 1/3 cup olive oil, pinch of salt, pepper, 1/4 tsp orange peel and garlic. Set aside.

Next, layer your dish.

First add your trimmed asparagus (or other vegetable of choice) and drizzle with olive oil or butter. Add a pinch (1/4 tsp or so) of lemon pepper seasoning.

Place your salmon (skin side down) on between the asparagus spears.

Drizzle the orange rosemary marinade on top of the salmon.

Add thin orange slices on top of the salmon and on top of the asparagus.

Place 2 to 2 fresh sprigs of rosemary evenly on top of the salmon and around the pan.

Sprinkle a bit more orange peel, pepper, and kosher salt on top of the salmon veggie bake.

Bake at 400F for 12-15 minutes or until salmon is not longer opaque in the middle.

Per serving: 345 calories, 22 g fat (3 g sat), 25 g protein, 10 g carb, 5 g sugars, 3 g fiber

Mushroom and Black Bean Smothered Burritos

Ingredients:

100 g (~ 1/3 cup) white rice

1 Tbsp oil

1 medium onion, sliced or diced

8 medium mushrooms, sliced or diced

2 cloves garlic, minced

2 tsp smoked paprika

1 tsp ground cumin

1 Tbsp tomato puree / paste

145 g (~ 2/3 cup) cooked black beans (~ 3/4 of a standard tin

Salt

Black pepper

4 large flour tortillas

150 g cheddar cheese, grated (~ 1 1/2 cups when grated)

1 Tbsp pickled jalapeños (I used green), finely chopped

1 Tbsp coriander (cilantro), finely chopped

3 Tbsp sour cream

Toppings, to serve (optional): diced tomatoes, diced red onion, black olives, fresh coriander, jalapeños, diced avocado, etc.

Directions:

Boil the rice in plenty of water until just cooked, then drain.

Meanwhile, heat a dash of oil in a large frying pan, and add the onion and mushrooms. Cook for a few minutes over a medium heat until slightly softened, then add the garlic, smoked paprika, cumin and tomato puree. Cook for a few more minutes, stirring regularly.

Add the black beans and the cooked rice, and season generously. Mix well to combine.

Take one of the large flour tortillas, and add about 1/4 of the rice mixture to the centre. Top with 1/4 of the grated cheese. Fold two sides of the tortilla inwards, then rotate through 90° and fold in the other two sides to fully wrap the burrito.

Repeat with the remaining tortillas, rice, and cheese, and place the burritos seam-side down on a baking tray.

In a small bowl, combine the finely chopped jalapeños, coriander, and sour cream. Season with a pinch of salt and pepper, and mix well.

Divide the sour cream sauce over the 4 burritos, and spread it around a little. Bake at 375 degrees F for around 15-20 minutes, or until crisped up to your liking. Serve with your choice of toppings.

Per serving: 486 calories, 22 g fat (10.7 g sat), 18.7 g protein, 53 g carb, 665 mg sodium, 3 g sugars, 5.4 g fiber

ARROZ CON POLLO, LIGHTENED UP

Ingredients:

8 skinless chicken thighs

1 Tbsp vinegar

2 tsp Sazon, homemade or Badia Sazon Tropical

about 1/2 tsp adobo powder, Goya

about 1/2 garlic powder

3 tsp olive oil

1/2 onion

1/4 cup cilantro

3 cloves garlic

5 scallions

2 Tbsp bell pepper

1 medium vine tomato, diced

2 1/2 cups enriched long grain white rice

4 cups water

1 chicken bouillon cube

kosher salt to taste, about 2 tsp

Directions:

Season chicken with vinegar, 1/2 tsp sazon, adobo and garlic powder and let it sit 10 minutes.

Heat a large deep heavy skillet on medium, add 2 tsp oil when hot.

Add chicken and brown 5 minutes on each side. Remove and set aside.

Place onion, cilantro, garlic, scallions and pepper in mini food processor. Add remaining teaspoon of olive oil to the skillet and sauté onion mixture on medium-low until soft, about 3 minutes.

Add tomato, cook another minute. Add rice, mix well and cook another minute.

Add water, bouillon (be sure it dissolves well) and remaining sazon, scraping up any browned bits from the bottom of the pot.

Taste for salt, should taste salty enough to suit your taste, add more as needed.

Add chicken and nestle into rice, bring to a boil. Simmer on medium-low until most of the water evaporates and you see the liquid bubbling at the top of the rice line, then reduce heat to low heat and cover. Make sure the lid has a good seal, no steam should escape (You could place a piece of tin foil or paper towel in between the lid and the pot if steam escapes).

Cook 20 minutes without opening the lid. Shut heat off and let it sit with the lid on an additional 10 minutes (don't peek!) Fluff with a fork and eat!

Per serving: 410 calories, 8 g fat (2 g sat), 33.5 g protein, 47 g carb, 655 mg sodium, 0.5 g sugars, 1 g fiber

Healthy Greek Chicken and Farro Salad

Ingredients:

1 1/4 cup quick-cooking farro

2 Tbsp olive oil

1/2 small red onion, thinly sliced

4 Tbsp lemon juice

Kosher salt and pepper

12 oz boneless, skinless chicken breasts, sliced ½ inch thick

1/4 cup fresh dill, chopped

8 oz grape tomatoes, halved

1/2 seedless cucumber, cut into ½-inch pieces

3 oz baby arugula (about 3 cups)

3 oz feta, crumbled

Directions:

1. Cook farro per package directions, then drain, transfer to a large bowl, and toss with 1 Tbsp oil.

2. Meanwhile, in a bowl, toss onion with 2 Tbsp lemon juice and a pinch of salt. Let sit, tossing twice.

3. Heat remaining Tbsp oil in a large skillet on medium-high.

Season chicken with ¼ tsp each salt and pepper and cook until golden brown, 8 to 10 minutes.

4. Remove the skillet from heat and stir in remaining 2 Tbsp lemon juice.

5. Add chicken and any juices to farro along with dill, tomatoes, cucumber, and onion (and their juices); toss to combine. Fold in arugula and feta.

Per serving: 380 calories, 10 g fat (1.5 g sat), 26 g protein, 198 mg sodium, 44 g carb, 4 g sugar (0 g added sugar), 7 g fiber

INSTANT POT BEEF AND BARLEY STEW

Ingredients:

1 lb beef chuck, well trimmed, cut into 2-inch pieces

1 Tbsp all-purpose flour

1 Tbsp olive oil

1 large onion, chopped

4 cloves garlic, smashed

8 sprigs thyme, plus leaves for serving

Kosher salt and pepper

1 12-oz bottle beer

1/2 medium butternut squash (1 pound), peeled and seeded, cut into 2-inch pieces

3 medium carrots (about 12 ounces), sliced

3 cup no-salt-added beef broth

1 cup pearled barley

Directions:

1. Set Instant Pot to sauté. In a medium bowl, toss beef with

flour. Add olive oil to Instant Pot, then cook beef until browned on all sides, 5 to 6 minutes. Transfer beef to a plate.

2. Add onion, garlic, thyme sprigs, and 1/2 teaspoon each salt and pepper and cook, stirring occasionally, until tender, 5 to 6 minutes. Stir in beer. Press cancel.

3. Return beef to pot along with squash, carrots, beef stock, and barley. Lock the lid and cook on high pressure 16 minutes. Use quick-release method to release pressure. Serve sprinkled with additional thyme if desired.

Per serving: 485 calories, 9 g fat (2 g sat), 35 g protein, 490 mg sodium, 67 g carb, 13 g fiber

Coconut-Lime Marinated Shrimp + Voodles

Ingredients:

3 limes

3/4 cup light coconut milk

1 tsp low-sodium soy sauce

2 cloves garlic

1 1-inch piece fresh ginger

1 red chile

1 1/2 cup fresh cilantro

2 scallions, thinly sliced, white and green parts separated

1 large, thick carrot

2 medium zucchini

1 red pepper, thinly sliced

1 lb cooked, peeled, deveined shrimp

Directions:

Finely grate zest of one lime into a large bowl, then squeeze in juice of all limes (should yield about 1/4 cup). Whisk in coconut milk and soy sauce. Finely grate in garlic, ginger, and 1/2 red chile. Finely chop 1/2 cup cilantro and stir into the bowl along with scallion whites. Thinly slice rest of chile and set aside.

Using a spiralizer fitted with the finest noodle blade, spiralize carrot, then use a larger blade to spiralize zucchini. Toss voodles in coconut milk mixture; let sit for 10 minutes.

After 10 minutes, fold in red pepper, shrimp, and remaining cilantro. Sprinkle with remaining scallions and sliced chile.

Per serving: 225 calories, 5.5 g fat (2.5 g sat), 32 g protein, 415 mg sodium, 14 g carb, 7 g sugars, 3 g fiber

Grilled Watermelon + Steak Salad

Ingredients:

1 lb sirloin (about 1 inch thick)

Kosher salt and pepper

3 Tbsp fresh lemon

2 Tbsp olive oil

2 tsp honey

1/2 small red onion, thinly sliced

1 lb cherry tomatoes, halved

1/2 small seedless watermelon

1 c. fresh mint, leaves torn

1 c. fresh flat-leaf parsley leaves

1 small bunch arugula, thick stems discarded

Directions:

Heat grill to medium-high. Season steak with 1/2 tsp each salt and pepper and grill to desired doneness (six to eight minutes per side for medium-rare). Transfer to a cutting board and let rest before slicing.

Meanwhile, in a bowl, whisk together lemon juice, oil, honey, and a pinch each salt and pepper. Fold in onion and tomatoes.

Cut watermelon into 1/2-inch-thick triangles and cut off rinds. Brush lightly with oil, then grill until lightly charred, one to two minutes per side. Divide among four plates.

Fold herbs into tomato mixture, then gently toss with arugula. Spoon on top of watermelon and serve with steak.

Per serving: 361 calories, 18 g fat (4.5 g sat), 28 g protein, 346 mg sodium, 24 g carb, 16 g sugar, 4.5 g fiber

SMASHED PEA AND RICOTTA PAPPARDELLE

Ingredients:

12 oz pappardelle

1 1/2 c. frozen peas, thawed

1 tsp lemon zest

1/2 c. part-skim ricotta cheese

1/2 tsp kosher salt

1/2 tsp pepper

1/4 c. chives, chopped

Directions:

Cook pasta per package directions. Reserve 1/2 cup cooking water; drain pasta and return to pot.

While pasta is cooking, pulse one cup thawed peas in a food processor until roughly chopped. Add zest and ricotta and pulse a few times to combine, then season with salt and pepper.

Toss pasta with ricotta mixture and remaining 1/2 cup peas, adding reserved pasta water if pasta seems dry. Sprinkle with chopped chives and serve.

Per serving: 430 calories, 6.5 g fat (2.5 g sat), 19 g protein, 100 mg sodium, 70 g carbs, 5 g fiber

Grilled Chicken with Smoky Corn Salad

Ingredients:

4 6-oz boneless, skinless chicken-breast halves

Salt and Pepper

2 limes, halved

4 ears corn, shucked

1/4 c. cilantro, chopped

2 tbsp. chopped green olives

1 oz. Manchego cheese, finely grated

1 1/2 tsp. olive oil

1 tsp. smoked paprika

Directions:

Season boneless, skinless chicken-breast halves with salt and pepper and grill on medium-high to cook through, 5 to 6 minutes per side.

Meanwhile, grill limes, cut sides down, and corn until charred, 6 to 8 minutes.

Cut corn from cob and toss in bowl with juice of 2 lime halves, then chopped cilantro, chopped green olives, grated Manchego cheese, and pinch each salt and pepper.

Serve chicken with corn and remaining lime halves and drizzle with a mixture of olive oil and smoked paprika.

Per serving: 355 calories, 13 g fat (3.5 g saturated), 21 g protein, 315 mg sodium, 21 g carb, 2 g fiber

WHITE BEAN AND TUNA SALAD WITH BASIL VINAIGRETTE

Ingredients:

Kosher salt and pepper

12 oz. green beans, trimmed and halved

1 small shallot, chopped

1 c. lightly packed basil leaves

3 tbsp. olive oil

1 tbsp. red wine vinegar

4 c. torn lettuce

1 15-oz can small white beans, rinsed

2 5-oz cans solid white tuna in water, drained

4 soft-boiled eggs, halved

Directions:

Bring a large pot of water to a boil. Add 1 tablespoon salt, then green beans, and cook until just tender, 3 to 4 minutes. Drain and rinse under cold water to cool.

Meanwhile, in a blender, puree shallot, basil, oil, vinegar, and 1/2 teaspoon each salt and pepper until smooth.

Transfer half of dressing to large bowl and toss with green beans. Fold in lettuce, white beans, and tuna and serve with remaining dressing and eggs.

Per serving: 340 calories, 16.5 g fat (3 g saturated), 31 g protein, 770 mg sodium, 24 g carb, 8 g fiber

Rhubarb and Citrus Salad with Black Pepper Vinaigrette

Ingredients:

2 tbsp. honey

2 tbsp. white wine vinegar

3 stalks rhubarb, trimmed and cut into 1-in. pieces

1/4 c. olive oil

Kosher salt and pepper

2 Cara Cara oranges

3 oz. baby spinach (about 4 c.)

2 bunches watercress, thick stems removed

1/4 c. toasted pistachios, chopped

1 oz. ricotta salata, shaved

Directions:

In small bowl, whisk together honey and vinegar. Add rhubarb and toss to coat. Let stand at least 5 minutes and up to 10 minutes, then add olive oil, 1/2 teaspoons salt and 2 teaspoons coarsely ground pepper.

Meanwhile, cut away peel and white pith from oranges, then thinly slice.

In large bowl, toss spinach and watercress; fold in orange slices and divide among plates. Spoon rhubarb and dressing over each salad and top with pistachios and ricotta salata.

Per serving: 280 calories, 19.5 g fat (3.5 g saturated), 5 g protein, 380 mg sodium, 25 g carbohydrate, 4 g fiber

Pot Sticker Stir-Fry

Ingredients:

Package of vegetable pot stickers or pierogies

2 tbsp. hoisin sauce

2 tbsp. fresh lime juice

1 tbsp. water

1 tbsp. vegetable oil

1 red pepper, thinly sliced

1 yellow pepper, thinly sliced

1 tbsp. finely chopped fresh ginger

1 small red onion, thinly sliced

8 oz. snow peas, halved diagonally

Directions:

Pan-fry vegetable pot stickers or pierogies in large skillet per package directions; transfer to plate. Whisk together hoisin sauce, fresh lime juice, and water.

Add vegetable oil to skillet and heat on medium. Add red pepper, yellow pepper, and finely chopped fresh ginger and cook, tossing frequently, 5 minutes. Add small red onion and cook, tossing, 1 minute.

Add snow peas and cook, covered, tossing often, until vegetables are just tender, about 4 minutes. Toss vegetables with sauce and serve with pot stickers.

Per serving: 240 calories, 6.5 g fat (0.5 g saturated fat), 7 g protein, 510 mg sodium, 41 g carb, 5 g fiber

Grilled Basil Chicken and Zucchini

Ingredients:

1 c. white rice

1 lime, plus wedges for serving

2 cloves garlic

1 tbsp. low-sodium soy sauce

1/2 tsp. sugar

1/2 red chile, thinly sliced

4 small zucchini (about 1 1/4 lbs), halved lengthwise

2 tbsp. olive oil, divided

Kosher salt and pepper

1 lb. chicken tenders

2 1/2 c. basil, roughly chopped

Directions:

Cook rice per package directions.

Zest lime into large bowl, then squeeze in 2 tablespoons juice. Finely grate garlic into bowl, then stir in soy sauce, sugar, and chile.

Brush zucchini with 1 tablespoon oil and season with 1/4 teaspoon each salt and pepper. Rub chicken tenders with remaining tablespoon oil and season with 1/4 teaspoon each salt and pepper. Grill zucchini until just barely tender and chicken until just cooked through, about 3 minutes per side; transfer to cutting board.

Cut zucchini and chicken into pieces and toss in sauce; fold in basil and serve over rice with lime wedges.

Per serving: 400 calories, 10.5 g fat (1.5 g saturated), 29 g protein, 450 mg sodium, 46 g carb, 3 g fiber

CHICAGO-STYLE CHICKEN DOGS

Ingredients:

2 jarred pepperoncini peppers, thinly sliced, plus 1 Tbsp brine

1 tsp. honey

1 tsp. yellow mustard, plus more for serving

1 tsp. poppy seeds

1/4 small sweet onion, thinly sliced

4 fully cooked chicken sausages

4 hot dog buns

2 small plum tomatoes, sliced into half-moons

4 dill pickle spears

1 small romaine heart, thinly sliced (about 3 cups)

Directions:

Heat grill to medium. In a bowl, whisk together pepperoncini brine, honey, and mustard; stir in poppy seeds. Add pepperoncini peppers and onion and toss to coat.

Grill sausages, turning occasionally, until lightly charred and heated through, 10 to 12 minutes. If desired, grill buns.

Stuff sausages into buns along with tomatoes and pickles. Toss poppy seeds and onions with romaine and spoon on top of sausages. Serve with remaining romaine mixture and extra mustard if desired.

Per serving: 490 calories, 16 g fat (3 g saturated), 18 g protein, 520 mg sodium, 66 g carb, 6 g fiber

Steak and Rye Panzanella

Ingredients:

2 tsp. caraway seeds

2 tbsp. red wine vinegar

4 tbsp. olive oil, divided

1 tbsp. whole-grain mustard

1 clove garlic, pressed

Kosher salt and pepper

1 bulb fennel, quartered

1 medium red onion, sliced into rounds

3 slices rye bread (1 inch thick)

1 large bunch kale, leaves chopped (about 10 cups)

1 lb. sirloin steak

Directions:

Toast caraway seeds in a small skillet on medium, about 2 minutes. In a small bowl, whisk together vinegar, 2 tablespoons oil, mustard, garlic, caraway seeds, and ¼ teaspoon salt.

Heat grill or grill pan on medium-high. Brush fennel, onion, and bread with 1 tablespoon oil and season fennel and onion with a pinch salt. Grill, covered, turning often, until vegetables are tender and charred and bread is toasted, 5 to 8 minutes for vegetables and 1 to 2 minutes for bread. Transfer to cutting board; core and thinly slice fennel and tear bread into chunks.

In a large bowl, toss kale, grilled vegetables, and bread with half of dressing and let sit, tossing occasionally.

Meanwhile, rub steak with remaining 1 tablespoon olive oil and season with ½ teaspoon each salt and pepper. Grill to desired doneness, 4 to 6 minutes per side for medium-rare. Transfer to cutting board and let rest 5 minutes before slicing. Fold into salad and drizzle with remaining vinaigrette.

Per serving: 435 calories, 23 g fat (5 g saturated), 29 g protein, 735 mg sodium, 28 g carb, 6 g fiber

CHEESY TEX-MEX STUFFED CHICKEN

Ingredients:

2 scallions (thinly sliced)

2 seeded jalapeños (thinly sliced)

1 1/4 c. cilantro

1 tsp. lime zest

4 oz. Monterey Jack cheese (coarsely grated)

4 small boneless, skinless chicken breasts

3 tbsp. olive oil

Salt

Pepper

3 tbsp. lime juice

2 bell peppers (thinly sliced)

1/2 small red onion (thinly sliced)

5 c. torn romaine lettuce

Directions:

Heat oven to 450°F. In bowl, combine scallions and seeded

jalapeños, 1/4 cup cilantro (chopped) and lime zest, then toss with Monterey Jack cheese.

Insert knife into thickest part of each of boneless, skinless chicken breasts and move back and forth to create 2 1/2-inch pocket that is as wide as possible without going through. Stuff chicken with cheese mixture.

Heat 2 tablespoons olive oil in large skillet on medium. Season chicken with salt and pepper and cook until golden brown on 1 side, 3 to 4 minutes. Turn chicken over and roast until cooked through, 10 to 12 minutes.

Meanwhile, in large bowl, whisk together lime juice, 1 tablespoon olive oil and 1/2 teaspoon salt. Add bell peppers and red onion and let sit 10 minutes, tossing occasionally. Toss with romaine lettuce and 1 cup fresh cilantro. Serve with chicken and lime wedges.

Per serving: 360 calories, 22 g fat (7.5 g saturated), 32 g protein, 715 mg sodium, 10 g carb, 3 g fiber

Herb-Roasted Chicken and Cherry Tomatoes

Ingredients:

1 tsp. plus 1 Tbsp oil

2 large bone-in chicken breasts (about 12 oz each)

3/4 tsp. salt

3/4 tsp. pepper

1 lb. cherry tomatoes (halved)

1 sprig rosemary

1 tsp. fennel seeds (crushed)

1 c. instant polenta

1 tsp. red wine vinegar

1/4 c. parsley (chopped)

Directions:

Heat oven to 450°F. Heat 1 teaspoon oil in large oven-safe skillet on medium. Season chicken breasts with 1/2 teaspoon each salt and pepper. Cook, skin sides down, until golden brown and crisp, 5 to 7 minutes.

Turn; add cherry tomatoes, rosemary and fennel seeds; drizzle with 1 tablespoon oil and season with 1/4 teaspoon each salt and pepper, then roast until chicken is just cooked through and tomatoes have begun to break down, 12 to 15 minutes.

Meanwhile, prepare polenta.

Discard rosemary; transfer chicken to cutting board and let rest 5 minutes. Stir red wine vinegar into tomatoes, then toss with parsley. Remove bone from chicken, slice and serve on polenta. Top with tomatoes.

Per serving: 445 calories, 17.5 g fat (4 g saturated), 32 g protein, 455 mg sodium, 37 g carb, 3 g fiber

. RED CURRY SHRIMP AND CILANTRO RICE

Ingredients:

1 c. long-grain white rice

1 tsp. grated lime zest

2 tbsp. fresh lime juice

1 c. cilantro (chopped)

1 tbsp. canola oil

1 1-inch piece ginger (cut into matchsticks)

2 cloves garlic (thinly sliced)

2 tbsp. Thai red curry paste

1 13.5-oz can light coconut milk

1 tbsp. fish sauce

1 1/2 lb. baby bok choy (4 to 6 heads, trimmed and leaves separated, large leaves halved lengthwise)

1 lb. peeled and deveined shrimp

Directions:

Cook long-grain white rice. Fluff with fork and fold in grated lime zest and cilantro.

Heat canola oil in large skillet on medium. Add ginger and garlic, and sauté 2 minutes.

Stir in Thai red curry paste and cook 2 minutes. Stir in light coconut milk and fish sauce and simmer 3 minutes.

Stir in baby bok choy and peeled and deveined shrimp and cook until shrimp are opaque throughout, 3 to 4 minutes. Stir in fresh lime juice. Serve over rice with additional cilantro, sliced red chiles, and lime wedges if desired.

Per serving: 405 calories, 11 g fat (6.5 g saturated), 24 g protein, 1,570 mg sodium, 51 g carb, 4 g fiber

Grilled Pork with Charred Harissa Broccoli

Ingredients:

2 lemons

1 1/2 lb. pork tenderloin

3 tbsp. plus 1 tsp olive oil

Kosher salt

Pepper

1 large head broccoli (about 1 1/4 lbs), trimmed and cut into large florets

2 tbsp. harissa

Directions:

Heat grill to medium-high. Finely grate zest of 1 lemon and set aside, then cut both lemons in half. Brush pork with 1 teaspoon oil and season with 1/2 teaspoon salt. Grill pork, turning occasionally, until it reaches 140°F on instant-read thermometer, 18 to 20 minutes. Transfer to cutting board and let rest at least 5 minutes.

Meanwhile, coat broccoli with 1 tablespoon olive oil and grill along with pork, turning often, until just tender and charred. Grill lemon until charred, 1 to 2 minutes.

Mix harissa with remaining 2 tablespoon oil and toss with broccoli; sprinkle with lemon zest.

Squeeze lemon halves over pork, then slice pork. Serve with broccoli and grilled lemon wedges.

Per serving: 330 calories, 16.5 g fat (3.5 g saturated), 38 g protein, 385 mg sodium, 8 g carb, 3 g fiber

NOOM LOADED SPAGHETTI

Ingredients:

1 cup sliced bell pepper

1/2 cup sliced red onion

1 tsp olive oil

1 cup cooked whole-wheat spaghetti

2/3 cup cooked edamame

Directions:

Sauté peppers and onions in oil until onions are translucent.

Toss with pasta and edamame.

Per serving: 420 cal

Cookout for One

Ingredients:

1 organic beef hot dog

1/2 cup organic baked beans

1 whole-wheat hot dog bun

1/2 Tbsp whole-grain mustard

1/2 Tbsp sweet relish

1 cup sliced honeydew melon

Directions:

Cook hot dog, and heat baked beans in a saucepan. Serve hot dog in the bun, topped with mustard and relish, with beans and melon on the side.

Per serving: 490 cal

Summer Farrotto

Ingredients:

1 boneless, skinless chicken breast (3 oz)

2 Tbsp olive oil, divided

1/4 cup sliced red onion

1 cup diced yellow squash

1/2 cup dry farro

1 Tbsp chopped parsley

1 Tbsp grated Parmesan cheese

Directions:

Pan-sear chicken in 1 Tbsp oil, seasoning with salt and pepper to taste, then dice.

Sauté onion and squash with remaining oil. Stir in farro until coated in oil. Add 2/3 cup water, bring to a boil, stir, reduce heat, and cover. Cook 20 minutes or until soft. Stir in chicken, parsley, and cheese, and serve.

Per serving: 490 cal

Beef and Veggie Salad Bowl

Ingredients:

2 Tbsp dry red quinoa

2 cups mesclun greens

3 oz cooked lean beef, cubed

1/2 cup chopped broccoli florets

1/4 red bell pepper, chopped

2 tsp olive oil

1 tsp red wine vinegar

Directions:

Cook quinoa as directed.

Toss with greens, beef, broccoli, and pepper in a bowl.

Whisk oil and vinegar for dressing.

Per serving: 320 cal

BOW TIES WITH SPRING VEGETABLES

Ingredients:

2 oz dry whole-grain farfalle pasta

2 tsp olive oil

1/2 cup artichoke hearts

1/4 cup sliced red onion

1/4 cup peas

1 Tbsp chopped fresh mint

Directions:

Cook pasta as directed and toss with oil, vegetables, and mint.

Season with salt and pepper to taste.

Per serving: 370 cal

Half-Homemade Soup with Asparagus

Ingredients:

4 oz boneless, skinless chicken breast

1 cup Amy's Organic Chunky Vegetable soup

2 Tbsp dry quinoa

1 cup chopped kale

10 small asparagus spears

2 tsp soy sauce

1/8 tsp grated fresh ginger

Directions:

Bake chicken at 350°F for 25 minutes, then shred with a fork.

Meanwhile, combine soup, quinoa, and kale in a saucepan, bring to a boil, and simmer until quinoa is done, about 15 minutes. Add chicken.

Steam asparagus, then toss with soy sauce and ginger. Serve asparagus on the side.

Per serving: 330 cal

Pork with Veggies

Ingredients:

1 pork tenderloin (4 oz)

1 cup steamed green beans

2 Tbsp sliced almonds

1 baked sweet potato

Directions:

Season pork with salt and pepper, sear in an ovenproof skillet coated with cooking spray, and transfer to a 450°F oven for 15 minutes.

Slice and serve with green beans topped with almonds, and a sweet potato.

Per serving: 370 cal

PIZZA PARTY

Ingredients:

1 Amy's Light 'N Lean Italian Vegetable Pizza

3 oz broccoli slaw

1/4 cup black beans

1/4 cup sliced scallions

1 tsp olive oil

1 oz lemon juice

Directions:

Bake pizza.

Blend slaw, beans, scallions, oil, and lemon juice, and serve on the side.

Per serving: 400 cal

Baked Chicken with Mushrooms and Sweet Potato

Ingredients:

1/2 skinless chicken breast

1 cup baby portobello mushrooms, sliced

1 Tbsp chives

1 Tbsp olive oil

1 medium sweet potato

Directions:

In a 350°F oven, bake chicken, topped with mushrooms, chives, and oil, for 15 minutes.

Microwave sweet potato for five to seven minutes.

Per serving: 382 cal

Shrimp Ceviche

Ingredients:

1/2 cup chopped cucumber

1/3 cup chopped jicama

1/3 cup chopped mango

1 Tbsp chopped onion

1/4 cup sliced avocado

1 tomato, sliced

1 cup cooked shrimp

1/4 cup lemon juice

1 tsp red pepper

Directions:

Toss together, and dress with lemon juice.

Per serving: 430 cal

Light Lasagna

Ingredients:

1/2 cup cooked whole-wheat spaghetti

1/4 cup part-skim ricotta

1/3 cup prepared tomato sauce

1/2 tsp crushed red chili flakes

1 Coleman Natural Mild Italian Chicken Sausage link, cooked

2 cups spinach

Directions:

Combine pasta, ricotta, sauce, and chili flakes, then crumble sausage on top. Add spinach, and let wilt.

Per serving: 350 cal

CHICKEN WITH CHEESY BROCCOLI SOUP

Ingredients:

1 cup chopped broccoli

1 cup chopped parsnips

3/4 cup nonfat chicken stock

1/4 cup low-fat shredded cheddar cheese

1 Tbsp sliced almonds

4 oz chicken breast

1 tsp lemon juice

Salt and pepper, to taste

Directions:

Steam broccoli and parsnips, then puree with stock and cheddar; sprinkle with nuts.

Bake chicken, top with lemon juice, and season.

Per serving: 360 cal

Cilantro Shrimp with Squash, Chard, and Wild Rice

Ingredients:

8 large shrimp

1 Tbsp olive oil

2 tsp fresh cilantro

2 tsp fresh lime juice

1 yellow squash, sliced

1 cup Swiss chard

1/4 cup dry wild rice blend

Sear shrimp in olive oil over medium heat for three to four minutes, seasoning with cilantro and lime juice.

Steam squash and chard for five to seven minutes, and cook rice according to package directions.

Per serving: 370 cal

Lemon Chicken with Gazpacho

Ingredients (chicken):

3 1/2 oz chicken breast

1 Tbsp olive oil

1/2 lemon, sliced

1 tsp fresh rosemary

Ingredients (gazpacho):

1 cup stewed tomatoes

3 cloves garlic, minced

1/2 cup onion, chopped

1/4 cup cucumber, chopped

1/4 cup green pepper, chopped

1 Tbsp white wine vinegar

Directions:

Coat chicken with olive oil. Cover with lemon slices and rosemary, and bake at 350°F for 25 to 30 minutes.

Combine gazpacho ingredients in a blender, then serve at room temperature with chicken.

Per serving: 414 cal

ZESTY TOFU AND QUINOA

Ingredients:

1 cup cooked quinoa

2 oz extra-firm tofu, cubed

3 Tbsp diced red pepper

3 Tbsp diced green pepper

1 tsp cilantro

2 Tbsp diced avocado

2 tsp fresh lime juice

Directions:

Combine all ingredients.

Per serving: 320 cal

Confetti Pesto Pasta

Ingredients:

1/4 pint cherry tomatoes

1/3 cup cooked green beans

1/3 cup diced chicken breast

1/4 cup pesto sauce

1/4 tsp each salt and pepper

1 cup cooked linguine

1/4 cup shredded Parmesan

Directions:

Combine tomatoes, cooked green beans, diced chicken breast, pesto sauce, and salt and pepper in a bowl. Add cooked linguine. Garnish with shredded Parmesan.

Per serving: 417 cal

Asian Turkey Lettuce Cups

Ingredients (turkey):

4 oz ground lean turkey

1/2 cup white mushrooms, chopped

1 tsp minced garlic

1/4 cup shelled and cooked edamame

2 Boston lettuce leaves

2 Tbsp sliced scallion

Ingredients (sauce):

1/2 Tbsp hoisin sauce

1 tsp low-sodium soy sauce

1/2 tsp rice vinegar

Ingredients (slaw):

1/2 cup shredded red cabbage and green cabbage

1/4 cup sliced jicama

1/4 cup grated carrot

1 tsp olive oil

1/2 tsp rice vinegar

Directions:

In a nonstick skillet coated with cooking spray, sauté first three ingredients for five minutes.

Add edamame, scoop mix onto lettuce, top with scallion, and wrap up. Drizzle with sauce, and serve slaw on the side.

Per serving: 329 cal

NOOM PORK WITH ROASTED VEGETABLES

Ingredients:

3 oz pork tenderloin

1 cup baked cubed butternut squash

2 cups brussels sprouts cooked in 1 Tbsp olive oil

1/2 tsp salt

1 tsp black pepper

Directions:

Roast pork tenderloin at 375°F, then serve with vegetables.

Per serving: 405 cal

Mushroom Bison Burger

Ingredients:

4 oz grass-fed bison burger

1 portobello mushroom, grilled

1 slice red onion

2 slices tomato

2 lettuce leaves

1 Arnold Artisan Ovens Multi-Grain Flatbread

Directions:

Grill mushroom and burger, and top with onion, tomato, and lettuce on flatbread.

Per serving: 374 cal

Salmon with Lemon and Dill

Ingredients:

5 oz wild Atlantic salmon

1 Tbsp lemon juice

1 tsp dill

2/3 cup parsnips

1 1/2 cup chopped broccoli, steamed

Directions:

Sprinkle salmon with lemon juice and dill and bake for 15 minutes at 225°F.

Per serving: 261 cal

Shrimp Pasta with Salad

Ingredients (pasta):

1/2 cup dry rigatoni, cooked

3 oz shrimp, poached

1/2 cup oil-packed sun-dried tomatoes, drained and pureed

3 large black olives, sliced

1/2 Tbsp pine nuts

2 tsp grated Parmesan

Ingredients (salad):

1 cup romaine lettuce

1/4 cup chopped tomato

1/2 cup sliced cucumber

1/2 Tbsp balsamic vinegar

Directions:

Toss pasta with shrimp, sun-dried tomatoes, olives, and pine nuts. Top with Parmesan. Serve alongside the salad.

Per serving: 465 cal

SEARED SCALLOPS WITH LEMON JUICE AND SAGE

Ingredients:

2 tsp canola oil

3 oz sea scallops

2 tsp lemon juice

1/2 tsp ground sage

1 1/2 cups cubed roasted acorn squash

2 cups kale sautéed in 2 tsp olive oil

Directions:

Heat canola oil in a large nonstick skillet over high heat. Add scallops and cook without stirring until well browned, around two minutes. Flip scallops and cook until the sides are firm and centers opaque, 30 to 90 seconds.

Drizzle with lemon juice, and sprinkle sage on top. Serve with squash and kale.

Per serving: 496 cal

Cheesy Veggie Pasta

Ingredients:

1/2 cup whole-wheat macaroni

1 cup crushed whole, peeled canned tomatoes

1/2 cup low-fat ricotta cheese

3/4 cup chopped spinach

1 cup zucchini wedges

2 tsp olive oil

Directions:

Cook vegetables over medium-high heat, then combine with cooked macaroni and cheese.

Per serving: 439 cal

Teriyaki Beef with Veggies

Ingredients:

3 oz grass-fed beef tenderloin, cubed

2 Tbsp reduced-sodium teriyaki sauce

1 Tbsp light honey-mustard dressing

2 tsp olive oil

1/4 cup sliced carrots

1/2 cup chopped broccoli

1/4 cup sliced water chestnuts

1/4 cup sliced peppers

1/2 cup cooked brown rice

Directions:

Marinate beef in teriyaki and dressing for 30 minutes.

Heat olive oil in a pan, and cook beef one to two minutes.

Add veggies, and cook for another five to seven minutes until beef is browned. Serve over rice.

Per serving: 506 cal

SHRIMP AND BROCCOLI PASTA SALAD

Ingredients:

4 oz cooked shrimp

1/2 cup cooked whole-wheat elbow macaroni

1/2 steamed broccoli

4 sun-dried tomatoes, halved

1 tsp capers

2 Tbsp red wine vinegar

1/4 tsp onion powder

1/2 tsp oregano

Directions:

Toss all ingredients, and serve cold.

Per serving: 312 cal

. Chicken Parmigiana with Penne

Ingredients:

4 oz grilled chicken, diced

1/2 cup tomato sauce

1 cup spinach

1/2 cup whole-wheat penne

1 1/2 Tbsp grated Parmesan

Directions:

Sauté spinach in one teaspoon olive oil, and toss with chicken, penne, and tomato sauce. Top with Parmesan.

Per serving: 437 cal

Beef Stir-Fry with Butternut Squash Soup

Ingredients (stir-fry):

3 oz steak tenderloin fillet, sliced thin

1/2 cup sliced shiitake mushrooms

1/2 onion, sliced

2 tsp olive oil

1/3 cup cooked bulgur

1/2 cup Pacific Natural Foods organic light-sodium butternut squash soup

Directions:

Stir-fry beef, onion, and mushroom, and serve over bulgur.

Per serving: 450 cal

Jambalaya Blend with Veggies

Ingredients:

1 veggie burger

1/2 cup cooked brown rice

2 Tbsp corn

2 Tbsp salsa

1/2 cup chopped red, green, or yellow bell peppers

3/4 cup diced squash

3/4 cup diced zucchini

1/4 cup chopped red onion

1 tsp olive oil

Salt, to taste

Directions:

Cook burger in pan spritzed with cooking spray, then chop burger and combine with rice, corn, and salsa.

Toss veggies with oil and salt, roast for 15 to 20 minutes, and serve on the side.

Per serving: 360 cal

Cod with Rosemary Polenta and Beans

Ingredients:

3 oz cod

1 tsp chopped fresh parsley

Dash of salt and pepper

1/4 cup dry polenta

1/2 cup 1 percent milk

1 Tbsp pine nuts

1/2 tsp rosemary

1/2 cup cooked green beans

Directions:

Season cod with parsley, salt, and pepper, then steam for eight minutes.

Cook polenta with milk, per package instructions, then top with pine nuts and rosemary. Serve with green beans.

Per serving: 352 cal

SHAVED ZUCCHINI SALAD

Ingredients:

2 medium zucchini, ribboned

1 cup halved cherry tomatoes

2 Tbsp pitted and chopped Kalamata olives

2 Tbsp diced feta cheese

1 Tbsp pine nuts, toasted

1 ½ Tbsp extra virgin olive oil

½ Tbsp apple cider vinegar

½ Tbsp balsamic vinegar

1 clove garlic, minced

¼ tsp freshly ground black pepper

Directions:

Combine oil, vinegars, garlic, and pepper in a small jar and set aside.

Add zucchini, tomatoes, olives, feta, and pine nuts in a bowl. Pour dressing over vegetables and cheese, toss to coat, and serve.

Per serving: 430 cal, 35 g fat (7 g sat), 26 g carbs, 15 g sugar, 610 mg sodium, 6 g fiber, 10 g protein.

JALAPEÑO-WATERMELON SALAD

Ingredients:

3 Tbsp extra virgin olive oil

1 Tbsp apple cider vinegar

1 Tbsp balsamic vinegar

1 clove garlic, minced

½ tsp salt

¼ tsp freshly ground black pepper

3 c arugula

2 c diced seedless watermelon

½ c halved cherry tomatoes

¼ c diced red onion

2 Tbsp diced feta cheese

2 Tbsp minced fresh mint

1 Tbsp seeded and minced jalapeño

Directions:

Combine olive oil, vinegars, garlic, salt, and pepper in a large bowl. Whisk until emulsified.

Add the arugula, watermelon, tomatoes, onion, feta, mint, and jalapeño. Toss with your hands to combine well. Serve immediately.

Per serving: 200 cal, 16 g fat (3 g sat), 13 g carbs, 9 g sugar, 470 mg sodium, 1 g fiber, 3 g protein.

Eggplant Parmesan

Ingredients:

1 large eggplant

2 zucchini

2 Tbsp olive oil, plus more for roasting vegetables

1/4 tsp sea salt

1 cup low-fat mozzarella

1 cup freshly grated Parmesan, divided

1/4 cup chopped fresh oregano

3/4 cup quinoa

1/4 cup chia seeds

1/4 cup fresh basil

1/4 tsp freshly ground pepper

1 jar marinara sauce (24 oz), no added salt or sugar

2 cups fresh spinach

Directions:

Peel the eggplant and zucchini and slice. Brush both sides with oil and arrange on a baking sheet. Sprinkle with salt and roast in a 400°F oven until tender, about 12 to 14 minutes.

Combine mozzarella, half the Parmesan, and oregano. Separately, mix quinoa, chia, remaining Parmesan, 2 tablespoons oil, basil, and pepper.

Spread half the marinara in a baking dish. Layer with half the vegetables, spinach, and cheese-oregano mixture. Repeat. Top with quinoa blend and bake for 25 to 30 minutes. Serves six.

Per serving: 350 cal, 18 g fat (5g sat), 33 g carbs, 11 g sugar, 510 mg sodium, 8 g fiber, 18g protein.

SPAGHETTI AND MEATBALLS

Ingredients:

1 lb lean ground turkey

1 cup cooked farro

1 cup spinach leaves

4 egg whites

4 Tbsp chopped onion

1 tsp oregano

1 tsp turmeric

Pinch of salt and pepper

4 sweet potatoes

4 Tbsp grated Asiago cheese

Directions:

Preheat oven to 350°F.

To make meatballs, mix together the first eight ingredients by hand, then roll into 16 balls, each about 1 inch in diameter. Place the balls on a sheet pan lined with parchment paper. Bake for about 30 minutes, or until golden brown on top.

Meanwhile, wash and peel sweet potatoes. Then, using the peeler, make thin ribbons from the flesh of the potatoes. Blanch ribbons in boiling salted water, then drain.

Serve meatballs atop the ribbons, sprinkled with grated Asiago. Serves four.

Per serving: 330 cal, 4 g fat (1.5 g sat), 38 g carbs, 6 g sugar, 260 mg sodium, 6 g fiber, 37 g protein.

Sweetgreen Portobello, Squash, and Wild Rice Bowl with Ginger Miso Dressing

Ingredients (bowl):

2 cups cooked wild rice, warm

4 cups kale leaves, shredded

1 handful basil leaves, torn

3 Portobello mushrooms, stemmed, diced, and roasted

1 small butternut squash, peeled, diced, and roasted

1 small red onion, peeled, diced, and roasted

1 medium red beet, peeled and diced

Ingredients (dressing):

2 Tbsp sweet white miso paste

2 Tbsp tamari or soy sauce

1 Tbsp sriracha (optional)

2 Tbsp rice vinegar

½ tsp sesame oil

¼ cup warm water

2 Tbsp mirin

1 thumb-sized piece of ginger, peeled and minced

1 garlic clove, smashed and minced

½ cup grape seed oil

Directions:

Combine all dressing ingredients except grape seed oil in a blender on low until smooth. Increase speed to medium while adding grape seed oil. Set aside.

Combine all of the salad ingredients in a large mixing bowl, and toss with your preferred amount of dressing. Serve immediately. Serves six to eight.

Per serving: 455 cal

EGGPLANT AND ZUCCHINI LASAGNA

Ingredients:

1 Tbsp olive oil

2 garlic cloves, minced

1/4 white onion, diced

1 can (28 oz) whole tomatoes, drained

2 cups ricotta cheese

Zest of 1/2 lemon

6 basil leaves, chopped, plus more for serving

3 parsley sprigs (leaves only), chopped

1 small eggplant, thinly sliced

1 small zucchini, thinly sliced

8 oz fresh part-skim mozzarella, sliced

Directions:

In a cast-iron pan on medium high, heat the oil, garlic, and onion, 3 to 5 minutes.

Add the tomatoes; stir occasionally till thickened, 5 to 10

minutes.

In a large bowl, mix the ricotta, zest, and herbs; season with salt and pepper. Spoon out half the sauce; set aside.

Now do layers in the pan: half the vegetables; half the ricotta mix; repeat; the rest of the sauce; mozzarella.

Bake in a 400°F oven, lid on, till tender, 20 to 30 minutes. Uncover and bake till the cheese is bubbly, another 5 to 10 minutes. Serves six.

Per serving: 313 calories, 20 g fat, 16 g carbs, 4 g fiber, 21g protein.

Printed in Great Britain
by Amazon